BEING HEALTHY CAN BE MADE EASY.

IT BEGINS WITH COMMON SENSE ALONG WITH PRACTICAL KNOWLEDGE.

THIS BOOK HAS BOTH.

DISCOVER THE REAL TRUTH!

Kaptur Press
1548 Adams, Suite D
Costa Mesa, California 92626

Note:

This book is designed to provide accurate and authoritative information on health. It is published with the understanding that neither the author nor publisher are engaged in rendering medical services. No attempt is made to diagnose or treat health conditions. If expert assistance is required, the services of a competent professional should be sought.

Library of Congress Cataloging-in-Publication Data

Nelson, William J. (William John)
The real truth about health.

Bibliography.
Includes index.
1. Chiropractic—Popular works. 2. Health.
I. Title. [DNLM: 1. Chiropractic—popular works.
2. Exertion—popular works. 3. Health. WB 905 N432r]
RZ244.N45 1987 613

Library of Congress Catalog Card Number 85-082587

ISBN: 0-936987-01-4

First Edition June 1987

Order form for additional copies is located at the back of this book.

the real truth about health

THE BOOK THAT TAKES THE *WORK* OUT OF BEING HEALTHY

william j. nelson

Edited by
Charles W. Musey
and
Robert Dees
•
Illustrations by
Mark Lorenzen

Kaptur
Press
Costa Mesa, California

*"Relieving human suffering
and diffusing universal knowledge
is humanitarian."*

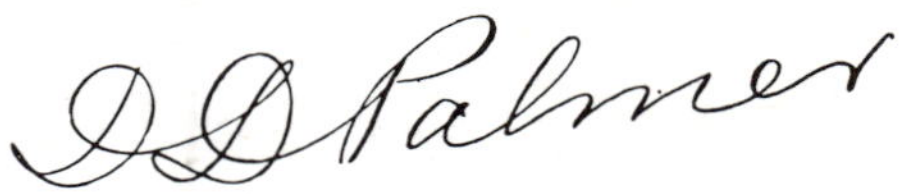

D.D. Palmer

Founder of Chiropractic

DEDICATION

To dedicate means to set apart for a definite purpose. For some, their purpose in life is obvious. Ultimately, all of us have a contribution to make. Countless numbers of people have touched me. I am indebted to the following for the significant contributions they made to my knowledge which is reflected in the information I am presenting.

To my Aunt Theresa, who shaped my attitude about ageing and the potential of the elderly: She taught me the basics of proper diet, introduced me to health food cooking, and kindled my interest in the pioneers of natural health. She drank bottled water in the early sixties, claiming that doing so would be commonplace someday. The test of a prophet is whether his or her words come true.

To Lisa Marie Shaft, whose death at an early age provided a sense of purpose and direction for others: Her life resulted in my continued exposure to innovative forms of health care.

To my grandmother, Helen Hattie Schultz: She possessed great strength of character. She was a simple person who showed that common sense could go a long way.

To my grandfather, Frank Day Nelson: He encouraged my inquisitive nature. As my first experience with someone dependent on life support systems, he intensified my search for the truth about health.

To Paul Bragg, N.D., R.Ph.T., a pioneer of natural health care and health food in this country: Bragg was living proof that people could have an almost ageless, painless, tireless body. He was vibrantly healthy into his nineties. His teachings on the subjects of diet, exercise, and internal cleansing are valid to this day.

To Hippocrates, the Father of Medicine and a great example of a medical practitioner: His ethics and philosophy have stood the test of time. His methods are preventive medicine at its best.

To Laurence Gallagher, D.C., a true follower of the methods of Hippocrates and Paul Bragg: Dr. Gallagher went out of his way to educate me about health. He felt health care needed more public input. He inspired me to learn with an open mind from as many sources as possible.

To Ben CiRullo, D.C.: Like Hippocrates, he is well versed in ethics, a very important aspect of life, especially as it pertains to health care. His relationship with me exemplifies what Confucius said: "When the student is ready, the teacher will appear."

To Burl R. Pettibon, D.C., who established a technique for understanding and adjusting the human spine as a precise science: Anyone can now be taught both the position and condition of the spine and thus learn how to specifically care for it.

Faith is the hardest of life's virtues to attain and maintain on a daily basis. Examples of its regular practice can be hard to find. I was fortunate enough to have two, my parents, Robert and Florence Nelson. I dedicate this book to them also.

ACKNOWLEDGEMENTS

My unreserved thanks to:
Charlie Musey, for editing and art direction.
Mark Lorenzen, for illustrations.
Robert Dees, for editorial guidance.
Louis P. Aguilar, Rochelle Clary, Rick Denman, Vern Gielow, Donald P. Hutchins, Tomas Kent, Xena Kistler, Kathleen Lanfried, Richard Lodyga, Joseph Martin, Patricia J. Mogan, Karen Reed, Cynthia Sedano, Leon Skeie, Daniel Tvedt, Robert van de Walle, and Alan White for their ideas and assistance. And to many others too numerous to mention for their support and suggestions.

WJN

ABOUT THE AUTHOR

William J. Nelson is a health care facilitator and fitness specialist, skilled and educated in health maintenance and disease prevention through application of basic health principles and common sense. His studies over the past ten years have fostered the creation of this work, ***THE REAL TRUTH ABOUT HEALTH***, and production of motivational workshops which he currently offers to both businesses and the general public.

As a researcher and journalist, Nelson has shared his acquired knowledge with thousands of individuals through his workshops and articles published in professional journals. His perspective of the health care field has enabled him to reduce its complexities to the essence and provide a broad scope of information.

The traumatic experience of watching his own father suffer the effects of a debilitating disease inspired him to seek out the truth about health. Nelson launched his career in a chiropractor's office initially as an assistant. He went on, however, to garner experience in all aspects of the business and application of health care, functioning as an office manager, X-ray technician, exercise therapist, public relations director, and facility administrator.

His education includes study of spinal bio-mechanics and engineering, anatomy, physiology, sports medicine, exercise physiology, and health care management and marketing. Extensive research into a number of health care disciplines has given him an intimate and wide-ranging perspective of care and maintenance of the body.

Driven by a thirst for knowledge and understanding, Nelson's research and education is on-going, as he continues to synthesize and translate health care information and discoveries into simple terms for the benefit of us all.

FOREWORD

Health care today is in an upheaval. One indisputable cause is the failure of doctors and patients to communicate effectively with one another. Yet it is difficult for a doctor to explain something to a person who lacks a common frame of reference. This book provides the framework of what patients should know. It will make doctor-patient relationships easier and more productive.

The author has extensive background as a health care administrator. He has been involved with every phase of operating a health care facility. Few people have such an intimate perspective about what goes on behind the scenes. He understands how different the perspective is for doctors, those who work for doctors, and most importantly, the consumer or patient. This book provides both theory and applications governing health care today. It comes from a unique perspective.

Nelson brings self-accountability to the forefront of the health care movement. His book contains the principles that form the foundation of knowledge regarding health. His simple methodology makes it possible to understand health on a personal level. It will ultimately provide people with greater physical self-understanding from which they can make enlightened decisions and take wise action.

Gordon H. Grannis D.C.

LIST OF ILLUSTRATIONS

Chapter 5

Chapter 6

Chapter 7

Chapter 8

Chapter 9

Chapter 10

CONTENTS

1

SEARCHING FOR THE TRUTH ABOUT HEALTH

"The preservation of health is a duty.
Few seem conscious that there is
such a thing as physical morality."

Herbert Spencer

I trace the beginnings of this book to two childhood experiences which significantly influenced my life. Through early exposure to the disasterous effects of my own father's physical illness, I learned at a young age the value of health and the importance of using common sense in maintaining it. By helping another take initiative to help his body fight illness, I learned that self-responsibility for the condition of one's own body is a necessary step to health.

I was born the last of four children, in a suburb of Detroit. My father, Robert Nelson, is of mostly Irish descent and was a carpenter by trade. My mother, Florence, is Polish on both her mother and father's side. We lived the American Dream as it was thought of in the 1960's. We had a home, a car, each other, and a bright future. But one day it all changed.

My father began having strange physical symptoms unlike those associated with a cold or flu. He was admitted to a local hospital where he underwent a battery of tests and examinations. The diagnosis was rheumatoid arthritis, a progressive constitutional disease characterized by inflammation and swelling of joint structures. He was only forty, my mother thirty-eight. I was four years old.

Rheumatoid arthritis extracts a slow death by robbing its victims of their strength. Simple body motion becomes painful and difficult. In 1962, little was known about how to treat my father's condition.

My brother Bob had to ease my father into the bathtub each morning with the help of pulleys and other devices. This hot bath eased the stiffness enough for him to function on his own. Then he would sit at the bathroom sink and soak his hands in hot paraffin wax. His pain was agonizing. Tears would roll down his cheeks each time he endured the experience. I will never forget how he suffered each day.

His being a carpenter didn't help my father's condition. He would come home from work exhausted and collapse after dinner. Even sleeping put pressure on his joints, waking him often. He had no escape from the disease or its pain.

His sickness changed the life and temperament of everyone in the family. The happiness we had known before was replaced by sheer day to day survival. Our belief in a secure and prosperous future vanished. As I saw my father's disease controlling my very existence, I began to realize my life would never again be the same.

My father was prescribed numerous drugs, so many in fact that his doctors had a hard time keeping track of them. He became a walking encyclopedia of pharmacology. As each drug failed to improve his condition, another took its place. The doctors tried everything available, hoping to find something that worked.

A couple of years later came cortisone, the wonder drug of the sixties. Labeled a cure-all for many ailments, it became our ray of hope. My father's disease was progressing at an alarming rate. Could cortisone stop its rampant and painful progression throughout his body? His survival—and to a large degree ours—depended on it.

At first, the cortisone seemed to work, and the disease went into a remission. My father's pain eased considerably, and he began to feel better. After a few months, he was working regularly again. But soon the dosage had to be increased as its effectiveness began to diminish. Although side effects developed, we still thought our prayers had been answered.

Within a year, serious side effects became evident. More tests were taken. The results were frightening. The cortisone had produced toxic effects which adversely affected my father's total physiology. His doctors wanted to discontinue its use, but a more serious problem had emerged. The drug was controlling the functioning of his thyroid gland. He would have to take cortisone the rest of his life and cope with the side effects. His body had become addicted to the drug.

Three years and several operations later, things had gotten worse instead of better. Dad grew weaker by the day. It was all he could do to go to work. He rarely went out, except to the doctor's or the hospital. I never knew from day to day what would happen next. My father's condition controlled our daily lives, keeping us on edge. I felt helpless and angry. There was no one to talk to about how unbearable it was to watch my father suffer. I loved him. He was an honest and hardworking man. Why him? I wondered. Why couldn't the doctors help him? We all had so much faith in them.

In desperation, his doctors tried gold shots, injections which actually contained a small amount of gold. They too, proved ineffective. He was also taking aspirin, fifteen to twenty or more a day to reduce the swelling of his joints. The drugs were overwhelming his body, which could no longer capably function on its own. He began taking drugs to counter the effects of other drugs. Finally, even the doctors became concerned about what the drugs were doing to him.

When I was thirteen, my father had to sell our house because he couldn't work full time anymore. Losing our home broke my parents' hearts. Life came to mean getting through the week with enough money to meet expenses and pay the doctor bills. Rarely would six months go by without my father being hospitalized. There were operations on the joints of his hands, his feet, his shoulders—virtually his entire body. The disease never let up.

We moved into a mobile home park. I felt confused and upset about my family's worsening situation and our strange, new environment. Anxiously, I set out to explore the neighborhood and make some new friends.

Our next door neighbors were in their late thirties, with a son, Mike, who was sixteen, and a daughter, Lisa, who was eleven months. They were outgoing, friendly, and progressive thinking people.

At one year of age, Lisa started having problems walking. Her doctors wanted to put her in braces. Her parents disagreed. What would happen when they removed them? Wouldn't she still have the problem? They thought putting braces on Lisa would amount merely to treating her symptoms. They wanted to find the cause of the problem and correct it. Their point of view made sense to me.

Her parents took Lisa to a chiropractor, who observed that her spine, possibly due to a fall, was out of its proper alignment. Over a period of several weeks, he adjusted Lisa's spine. Once her spine was properly re-aligned, Lisa's symptoms, the inability to walk properly, disappeared. To say the least, this turn of events fascinated me.

That treating causes was a better solution than treating symptoms was a revelation to me. I realized that none of the treatments rendered my father dealt with the condition and working operation of his spine. At that point, I began to understand certain aspects about health and its relation to human anatomy. Once I began learning about the brain and spinal cord, I recognized the tremendous role they play in a person's health.

THE BRAIN, SPINAL CORD, AND SPINAL COLUMN ARE YOUR BODY'S MOST IMPORTANT ORGANS

Without exception, the brain and spinal cord are the first organs created in every person. Together, they form the central nervous system, the master communication system of the body. For protection, they are the only organs encased in solid bone. The brain is encased in the skull or cranium, the spinal cord in the spinal or vertebral column. The brain communicates with the body through the spinal cord, which by spinal nerves branches out between the bones of the spinal column to every organ, tissue, and cell in the body. Along with the cranial nerves that arise from the brain, the spinal nerves form the peripheral nervous system. Though the spine is often referred to as one unit, the spinal cord and spinal column are two separate and distinct parts of the body (Figures 1.1, 1.2, 1.3, 1.4).

The basis of health starts with the spine. Hippocrates, the Father of Medicine, said, "Look well to the spine for the cause of disease" (Petersen 77).[1] The muscular and skeletal structures of the body rest upon the spinal column. Made up of twenty-four individual, moveable bones called vertebrae, along with the sacrum and coccyx, the spinal column surrounds the spinal cord

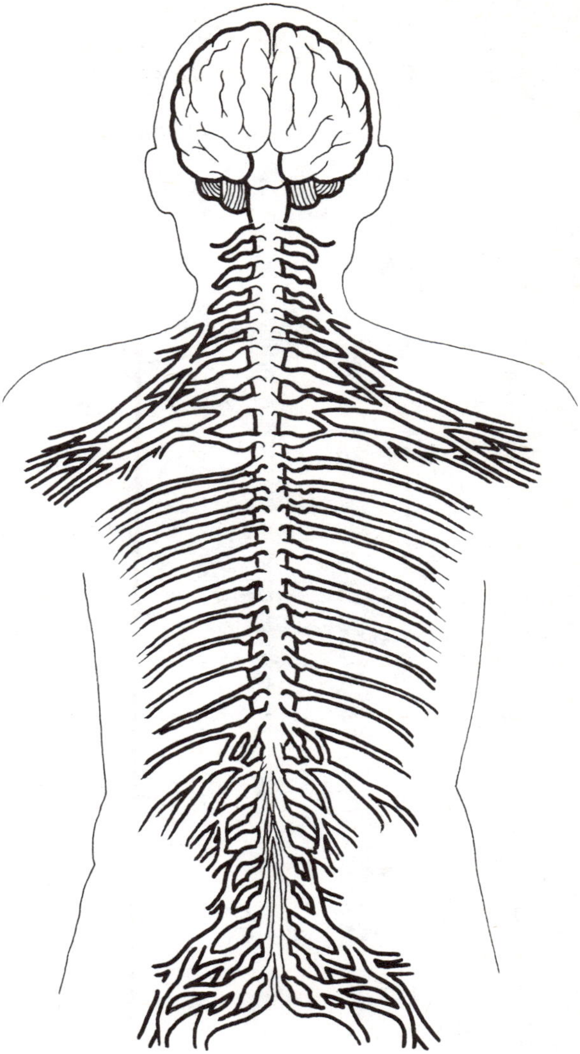

BRAIN AND SPINAL CORD

Figure 1-1

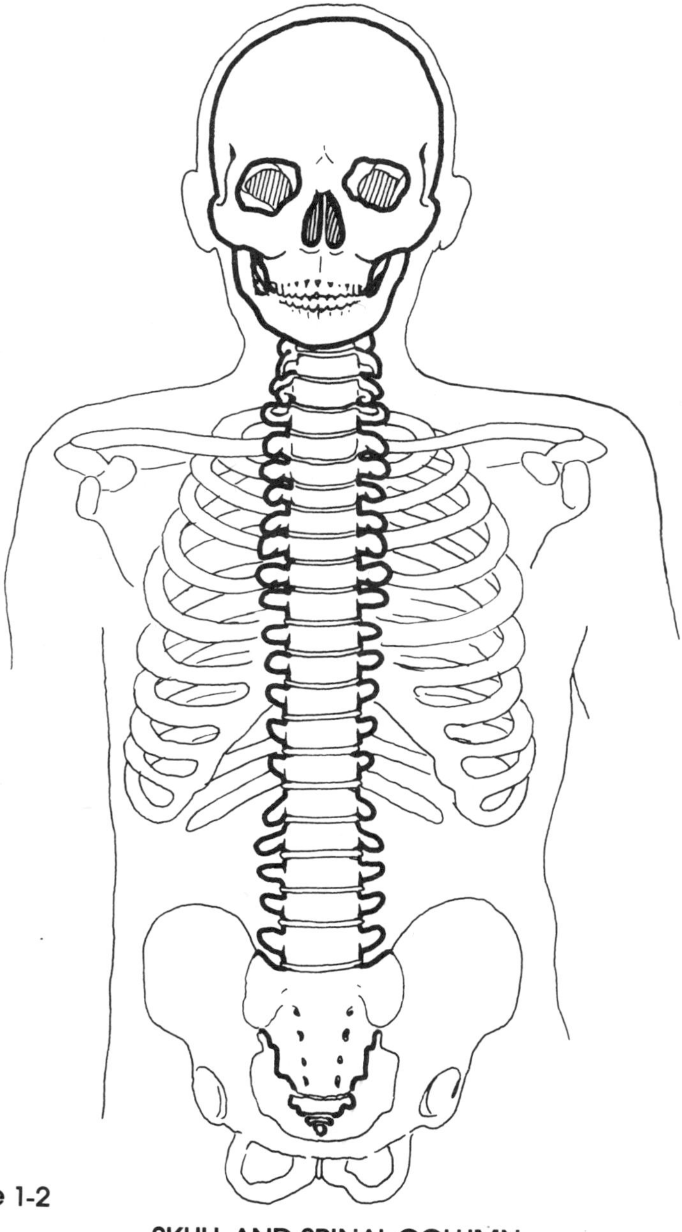

Figure 1-2

SKULL AND SPINAL COLUMN

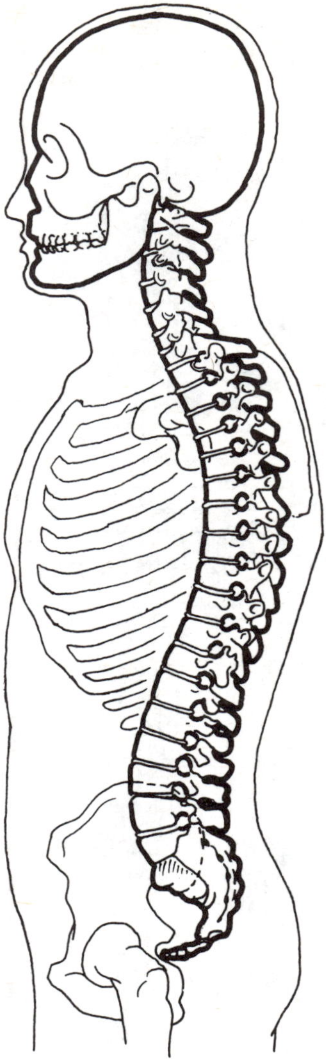

SKULL AND SPINAL COLUMN, SIDE VIEW

Figure 1-3

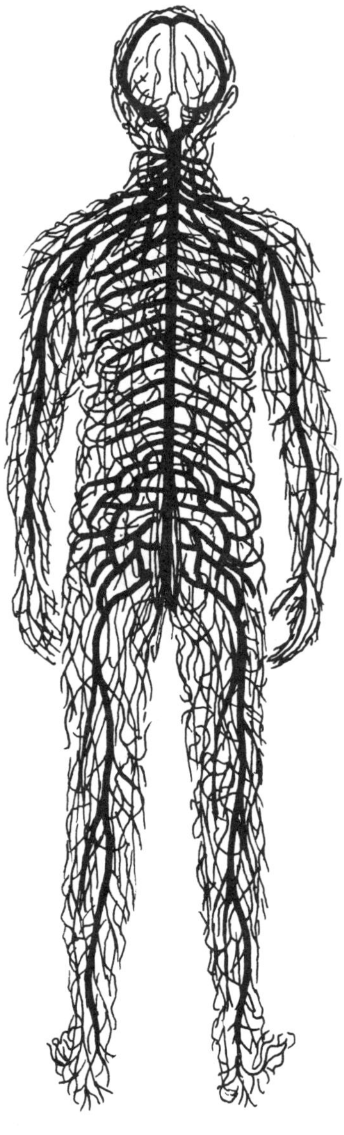

NERVOUS SYSTEM

Figure 1-4

with tightly connected walls of bone. Your spine is what supports you. Virtually all body motion originates at the spinal column, which itself must be in good working condition for free and unrestricted movement. In addition, it also absorbs the force and physical stress the body goes through every day.

I had wondered if a bad spine could be contributing to my father's problems. Watching him walk, it was obvious that his back was out of alignment. One hip was noticeably higher than the other, the result of an improperly set broken leg in childhood.

I once suggested to my father that he see a chiropractor, but his doctors had said chiropractors were quacks and that his back was fine. The doctors advised my father to continue with the treatments they had prescribed. Eventually, they signed papers declaring him totally and permanently disabled. At age fifty-two, he could no longer work, not even part time. He felt his life was over, that he might as well be dead.

By this time I was sixteen and continually exploring alternative methods of health care. It was becoming obvious to me that the spine played a vital role in a person's health. I wondered why this fact wasn't common knowledge.

A year later I suffered a concussion playing hockey. I was taken to the hospital, X-rayed, and examined for a possible skull fracture. Fortunately, no fracture was found. Yet no one made even a token attempt to see if my spine had been injured. After a month or so, I started getting headaches and had difficulty moving my neck freely. Soon, its range of motion became limited. Giving up on traditional treatment, I decided to go to a chiropractor myself and see firsthand what "quacks" did.

The chiropractor examined both my skull and spinal column. He explained the three main parts of the spine—cervical, thoracic, and lumbar. The cervical spine forms the neck and supports the skull. It comprises the top seven vertebrae (or bones) of the spine. These vertebrae form a natural curvature, giving the spine strength and leverage, allowing the neck to move freely.

X-rays showed that the trauma from my injury was so great it had straightened out my neck's natural curvature. More so, part of my neck was curved in the opposite direction, putting stress on the spinal nerves in that area.

With his hands, the chiropractor adjusted my neck by gently shifting the bones back to their normal positions. He prescribed exercises to strengthen my back and the neck muscles which keep the spinal column properly aligned.

This method approached health from a vastly different point of view than I had experienced before. I was eager to learn more about it. I soon realized that health was a combination of many factors and that the brain, spinal cord, and nervous system played important roles. Furthermore, I started to see that, to a large extent, each person had control over his or her own body and health.

Seeking to explore and experiment for myself, I started looking for other evidence of the spine's importance to health. In the high school library one day, I noticed a boy who could not stand up straight. He used a walker, dragging one leg and moving as much from side to side as forward. His name was Roger, and he had cerebral palsy. His disability was the result of brain damage caused by lack of oxygen at birth. From his posture, I could tell his spine was in poor condition.

Since Roger's voice was distorted, it took me awhile to understand him when we first met. I noticed that his right hand curled inward and that he had little use of it. Most of his muscles were atrophied, their movement restricted. He was as stiff as a board and greatly dependent on others for his daily care.

I knew that because of brain damage, Roger would never function normally. Despite his physical problems, he still maintained a positive outlook on life. But could his back, in its distorted configuration, be contributing to his condition? Could he ever be any better off than he was now? I concluded that only by working with Roger could I validate or disprove my thinking.

When I talked to Roger about going to a chiropractor, he laughed at me. None of his prior treatments had ever dealt with the condition of his spine. His doctors said there would never be much improvement. They considered his case closed. I disagreed. His back and overall condition could be improved, I insisted. I offered to drive him to the chiropractor's office, pay the bill, and help with any prescribed therapy. He resisted, but finally gave in to my persistence. Then I had to convince his family to go along with the idea.

At first, they too thought I was joking. When it became apparent I wasn't, they were downright angry. They had taken care of him his whole life. He had received the best medical care available. What qualified me to say Roger's condition could be improved? How dare I say his doctors had overlooked something—the doctors were the experts! But I disagreed. I had to test my theories, and Roger was the perfect case.

On our first visit, the chiropractor took X-rays. They were shocking. Roger's spine was severely distorted and appeared to have been that way for quite some time. Changing his spine's configuration would take a tremendous amount of effort, if it could be done at all. I thought I was in over my head.

The chiropractor had to work on Roger's spine daily for the first week and then three times a week for a month. Roger also required daily exercise therapy to loosen up and strengthen the muscles in his back. The doctor was willing to help all he could, even financially. He charged only a dollar per visit.

We went for several weeks without results. I became somewhat discouraged. Roger's family was convinced I was more of a quack than the chiropractor. Roger himself thought he was wasting his time and wanted to quit. Nevertheless, I persisted.

After three months, our efforts began to take effect. By exercising daily with my help, Roger gradually gained more control over the use of his body. Though he still needed support to stand, a cane in each hand replaced his walker. His right hand began to straighten. Now we saw the chiropractor only once a week. As Roger's legs got stronger, he started walking straighter, with less side to side motion. He developed more coordination. Week by week, his condition steadily improved.

At age nineteen, after fourteen months of effort, Roger walked by himself for the first time. I have never been filled with a greater sense of accomplishment. We couldn't wait to see the chiropractor to share the success of his chiropractic adjustments, physical therapy, and our hard work. For his new found abilities, Roger was especially grateful to the chiropractor.

I expected the chiropractor to float out the door on his ego. His remarks surprised me. He would take no credit for Roger's improvement. The chiropractor said he was a tool, nothing more. Our efforts had unlocked the innate healing potential of Roger's own body. It was that potential which produced the results.

Through this experience, I began to comprehend the great inner intelligence of the human body. The role it plays in health is vital and cannot be disregarded or circumvented. You can't live without it.

Searching for truth about health is a direct result of my childhood experiences. It is my mission. My findings, as they are expressed in this book, provide a basic foundation for understanding the components of health: self-responsibility, practical knowledge, and common sense. With that in mind and dedication on your part, you can take necessary action.

Telling you what to do with your body is NOT my intention. This book provides a starting point in understanding your body and what you can do to take care of it. I am presenting this material from a consumer's point of view.

Seeking and absorbing knowledge about health results in making intelligent health care decisions. This process can often be confusing. In order to make progress, my own experience has taught me the following logical steps to assimilate information about health and make use of it in my daily life.

THE SIX STEPS TO FACILITATE HEALTH

1. **OBSERVE**
2. **REFLECT**
3. **THEORIZE**
4. **EXPERIMENT**
5. **ANALYZE**
6. **COMMUNICATE**

OBSERVE what is going on in your life and the world around you. This is the act of gathering information. Collect from a variety of sources and points of view.

REFLECT on the information you have gathered. This is the process of contemplation. Decide what information is relevant and what is not.

THEORIZE about why things are the way they are and what you can do about them. This means consolidating your ideas into specific frames of reference. Allow yourself to compose creative solutions.

EXPERIMENT with various methods of solving your problem. This is the very important action part. Apply methods that your own observations tell you might work safely. Acknowledge that time is an essential element in any process involving the body.

ANALYZE your results. Find out if your solution stands up to scrutiny. Be honest and thorough. Use common sense.

COMMUNICATE your ideas and findings to others. This simply means sharing. Expect discussion and criticism. Keep in mind that what may apply to you may not necessarily be the answer for someone else. It is the *quality* of the process of searching for truth that counts.

This book is *not* the last word on the subject of health, nor will there ever be such. Recognize that as new data becomes available, we are required to re-evaluate prior beliefs and information. Every one of us can contribute to this body of knowledge. The six steps to facilitate health are meant to expedite the process. We all will gain by every effort put forth.

It is your responsibility to give your body the best care you can. An idea must immediately be put into action or it will lose the drive behind it. This book is one way to begin doing so now.

2

THE EVOLUTION OF HEALTH CARE

"The first wealth is health."

Ralph Waldo Emerson

The human race has studied and practiced health care for centuries. Many diligent seekers of truth have undertaken the quest for the sake of knowledge and the service of humanity. Others have pursued health simply for profit.

At the dawn of humanity, everything was open for discovery. Some questions surfaced early: Who am I? How did I get here? Where am I going? Philosophy and religion developed in order to answer those questions.

The establishment of certain strongly held beliefs started to consolidate people's way of thinking. Those adept at controlling people's spiritual needs gained tremendous social power. Power and prestige also went to those who could influence a person's health.

For centuries, people didn't know how the body actually functioned. Since no one knew what caused or cured illness, early healers tried everything. Trial and error was the only way to find out. If something worked, that information was in demand. Getting people well became a marketable commodity.

Early healers convinced people to believe in their advice, to follow it, and pay for it. Medicine was born, although its own identity took time to develop. Religion and medicine were thought of in the same context. There was little separation between the major studies of gods, the spiritual or supernatural, humanity, and the physical world.

Those who combined religion and medicine enjoyed great prosperity. Spiritual teachings were coupled with healing methods. The use of dramatics and witchcraft added excitement, mystery, and motivation. The practitioner of medicine at this time could be best thought of as a priest-healer.

As humanity evolved, knowledge expanded, and mastering one's vocation took more time. As vocations became more defined, greater separation grew between them. But for the most part, it would take centuries before a clear line of distinction between religion and medicine developed. Controlling the mind meant controlling the body as well.

About 600 B.C., a concept developed that defined humanity as two halves of a whole, therefore making mankind divisible. This was during the time of the Greek philosopher Theles, considered the Father of Philosophy. Thus began a new approach to the study of humanity.

The soul or spirit became one subject of study. The corporeal, material, and tissue structure became another. This belief, in essence, separated human beings into body and soul (B.J. Palmer *Philosophy* 6).[2]

As a result of such a philosophy, physicians assumed control over the physical body. The soul became the property of theologians. Each claimed exclusive rights to study and investigate their entity. As a result, religion and medicine solidified separate foundations and became part of the fabric of society. This separation consolidated power and control.

Consequently, individuals became less responsible for their own health and spirituality. Religious and medical practitioners, now given that responsibility, were paid well for their services. Additionally, they achieved a high level of social standing, a situation which is still true today.

As the practice of medicine developed, different schools of thought emerged. Over a long period of time, they solidified into two major philosophies. One philosophy advocated working in harmony with nature and the natural functions of the human body. In opposition, the other proposed taking control of the body. Some practitioners, following the former philosophy, utilized methods to help people better understand and care for their bodies. Others practiced medicine, following the latter philosophy, as a way to control their clients, transact business, and become wealthy.

The ancient Greeks were instrumental in developing medicine as an organized and ethical practice. A famous doctor of that time, and of all time, was Hippocrates, who lived from 460 B.C.

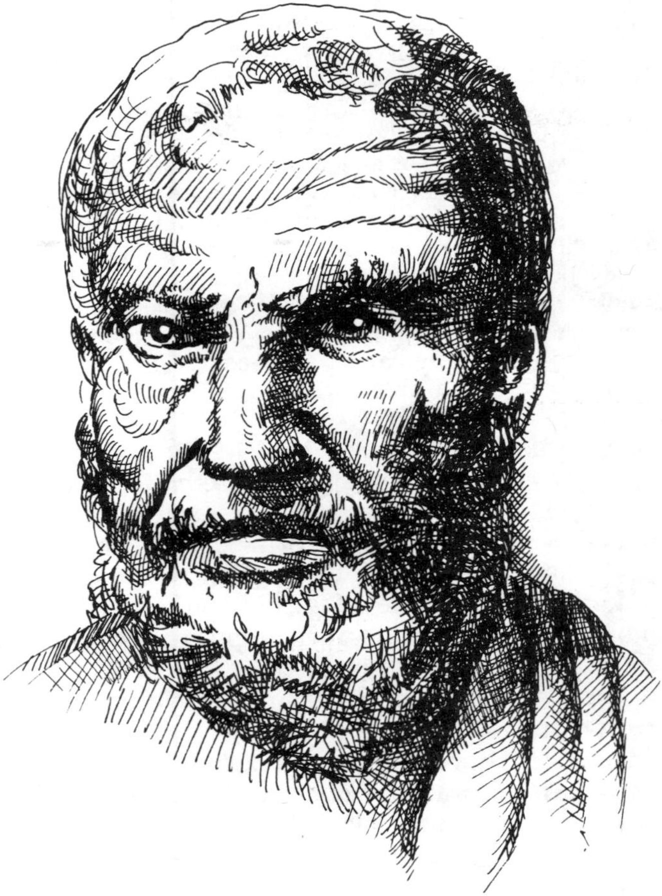

HIPPOCRATES

to 377 B.C. Considered the Father of Medicine, Hippocrates is remembered for his great humanitarian and professional skills, exemplary conduct, and noble views of the world. His high standard of professional ethics was impeccable.

His greatest impact on the medical profession, in fact, involved the espousal of professional standards of conduct along with moral principles and practice. The following is a modified version of the Hippocratic Oath:

> I solemnly pledge myself to consecrate my life to the service of humanity. I will give to my teachers the respect and gratitude which is their due; I will practice my profession with conscience and dignity; the health of my patient will be my first consideration; I will respect the secrets which are confided in me; I will maintain by all means in my power the honor and noble traditions of the medical profession; colleagues will be my brothers; I will not permit considerations of religion, nationality, race, party politics, or social standing to intervene between my duty and my patient; I will maintain the utmost respect for human life, from the time of conception; even under threat, I will not use my medical knowledge contrary to the laws of humanity. I make these promises solemnly, freely and upon my honor (Etziony 89).

Today, virtually every licensed medical doctor takes the Hippocratic Oath. It serves as the basis for ethical practice and service to humanity. Yet few physicians have actually been taught to follow Hippocrates' philosophy of medicine, which advocated working in harmony with the body rather than controlling it.

In addition to his code of medical ethics, Hippocrates is remembered today for another important contribution to medical practice, the concept of holistic healing. Hippocrates taught and practiced concern for the whole patient, not just afflicted organs.

Furthermore, Hippocrates realized that it wasn't the doctor who cured disease. Rather, an inborn force contained within a person's body was responsible for restoring health. To him, the duty of a doctor was to work in harmony with the inborn force and support nature's healing activities. This meant doing nothing that would infringe upon or disturb the natural process. The doctor's role was that of a helper only (Venzmer 79).

There were others who held similiar views. According to ancient Chinese pathology, illness was the result of alienation from the natural order of the universe. Similarly, doctors in early India focused attention on the prevention of illness as well as the cure. Other doctors, however, did not practice medicine in this manner.

The other emerging philosophy of medicine developed potions and treatments designed to elicit a physical change in the body. Changing a person's physical condition became the primary concern. This type of doctor believed every problem had a specific "cure." Healing was a matter of finding the right one without killing the patient in the process. Focus was placed on external or symptomatic changes in the body, thereby ignoring the totality of a person's condition. This methodology became the basis of their remuneration.

For the patient to believe in this method of treatment became highly profitable for the doctor. Seemingly miraculous cures brought in more payment. Too often, the doctor treated the symptom of the patient's problem, not the cause. This procedure was the exact opposite of Hippocrates' methods.

Hippocrates said, "Every illness, even though it may reveal itself by means of local symptoms, is nevertheless first and always a general disease and the individual part can never be recognized without seeing the whole" (Venzmer 75). He treated each patient uniquely, using his skills to work in harmony with the inner force of the patient's body.

Claudius Galenus, or Galen, a Greek physician and writer, born in Rome in AD 129, was an important early medical experimentalist. In Galen's time it was widely believed that evil spirits caused disease. The standards of the medical profession were lax, and many doctors had the sole aim of transacting business as quickly as possible, transferring their medical skill into financial gain. Furthermore, religious beliefs stifled scientific investigation by forbidding dissection of human corpses.

Though a highly skilled investigator, Galen was limited to the dissection of animals. Relating their anatomy to humans was erroneous. Despite this, Galen's work was highly respected and considered correct for more than a thousand years. The longer concepts such as these went unchallenged, the more medicine plunged into long, stagnant periods. During the Dark Ages these beliefs and practices impeded the search for the truth about health.

Almost fifteen hundred years after Galen, Andreas Vesalius (1514-1564), a Flemish anatomist and physician considered the Father of Anatomical Science, began to discover many falsehoods. Under the cover of darkness, Vesalius visited cemetaries and execution grounds, secretly unearthing recently buried bodies and dissecting them (Venzmer 142).

As Vesalius learned firsthand about human anatomy, he realized that Galen had never dissected human beings. Galen had erroneously applied to the human body, without seeing or checking, what he had found in animals (O'Malley 6).

Health care since Galen's and Vesalius' days has come a long way. We have overcome much of the ignorance, misinformation, and even the greed that hindered their own and their ages' search for truth, but we still have a long way to go. Part of our health care problem today stems from the attitude of individuals unwilling to be accountable for their own health. Doctors are thus put into the position of alleviating symptoms as quickly as possible. The result has been the development of an accepted system of administering crisis care.

CURRENT HEALTH CARE CONDITIONS

Hippocrates established the fact that the patient's body always does the healing and that the doctor is never more than a tool. Although modern medicine is highly advanced, the inner or innate healing force of the body still does the actual healing. Machines and medicines only assist this natural process. To be effective, the external forces must always work in harmony with the innate power of the body.

The innate power of the body is the controlling mechanism. It is the force that keeps one breathing, the heart beating, and food digesting without conscious thought. It handles all of the body's mechanical functions. The truth about health means living in harmony with that innate force.

Medicine and health care today is at once phenomenal, complex, brilliant, exciting, frightening, and expensive. Tremendous strides and growth have occurred in many areas. Doctors now have incredible resources available to them. Knowledge is abundant and ever growing concerning the workings of the human body.

Other sophisticated advances include artifical limbs, organ transplants, care of premature babies, and the use of life-support systems. Many of these advancements are a result of our space-age technology. Unfortunately, they also carry a hefty price tag.

There is a definite place for life-support systems. Unquestionably, they vastly improve emergency care and make seemingly impossible operations almost routine. Machines can keep us alive in cases when one would certainly have died in earlier days. But the situation is not utopian. The line of distinction between life and death continues to blur as time goes on. One can only speculate what those changes will impose upon the legal and moral areas of life.

The use of machines certainly can lengthen a person's life. But what about the quality of that life and the expense? Who wants to spend the last days of his or her life hooked up to machines? And where does the money come from to pay for these services?

THE COST OF HEALTH CARE

America's current expenditure for health care is rising dangerously high. Perhaps your own experience can verify this fact. Remember your last doctor bill? As health care costs increase, a greater portion of our resources (your money) is spent.

The total cost of our nation's health care is over 10% of the Gross National Product (Census 94). Average daily costs for health care in the United States are now over one billion dollars and rising (Census 96). How is that affecting our economy?

The high cost of health care is throwing our economy out of balance by consuming a disproportionate share of our disposable income. Many areas of health care have far surpassed the general inflationary rate (Almanac 51). As consumers, we pay for these increased costs: Taxes are increased to support Medicare and state-sponsored health care services. Health insurance premiums continue to rise, along with the costs paid by individuals, to cover what insurance does not. Salary increases are smaller to compensate for the increased cost of health insurance benefits paid by employers. Finally, private health care costs increase to offset what Medicare and other government programs fail to cover. We are paying more money directly out of our pockets as the government allocates less of its money (our tax dollars) to cover health care costs. Maybe the best illustration of our problems with this growing financial monster is that a major reason for personal bankruptcies in the United States today is catastrophic illness.

Ten percent of the entire yearly Medicare budget covers a patient's last year of life. Of that, a third goes for the last month of life (Nelson 1).

The health care industry is not fully to blame. The public has long avoided dealing with health care costs, feeling that medical care should be the right of each citizen. People want the best and most innovative care available, often not concerning themselves with cost. Health care is the only market commodity for which the person paying for it, the person using it, and the person providing it have an indirect rather than direct relationship.

Let's take a hypothetical example. John Doe is an employee. When he gets sick, he visits the doctor. The fees the doctor charges are paid for by John's insurance. The insurance is paid for by John's employer.

The employer is the person paying the bill. But the employer is not the recipient of the services rendered by the doctor. This situation means no one is directly accountable for the costs involved.

Employers do not directly dispense or receive health care. They have little control over it. Neither the patient nor the doctor are too concerned, because someone else (the employer) is paying for it. Many people falsely think that not having to pay the doctor bill means free medical care. Not so. Today, health care costs are a major portion of benefits provided to employees.

Costs rise because responsibility for the health of the patient is taken out of the patient's hands. Responsibility has been given to a third party, the health care provider, with a *carte blanche* expense account charged to the insurance company and paid for by the employer.

Without a direct line of accountability concerning expenses, the cost of health care spirals upward. The doctor has no incentive to charge less. Little money is received directly from the employee. Services are rendered to one party and paid for by another. The doctor and the patient make decisions without direct accountability for the cost.

Another important financial aspect of health care today is the number of lawsuits against doctors. Three times as many lawsuits are filed today in the United States than were filed ten years ago. Though many of these lawsuits are well founded, there is often a fine line between negligence on the part of the doctor and unforseen complications. Settlements for successful malpractice suits now reach exorbitant proportions, averaging over a quarter million dollars per case ("*Doctors on Defensive*" 188). Who pays for all of this? We do, in higher health care costs!

In response to the increasing number of lawsuits, doctors' malpractice insurance rates have increased 236% in the last ten years. Doctors in high-risk specialties often pay annual premiums of over $100,000 ("*Doctors on Defensive*" 188). These astronomical rates result in doctors increasing the amount of diagnostic testing, monitoring, and documentation to protect themselves from lawsuits, all of which adds unnecessary costs. But we are responsible for causing this situation as well.

Many of us have unreal expectations about medical services today. When something goes wrong, it's easy to blame the doctor. We must realize that as technology increases, so do the risks involved. It becomes increasingly difficult for doctors to become aware of and monitor the countless complications that can arise. They are often dealing with drugs and devices so powerful that it is almost impossible for even the most competent and conscientious doctor to accurately ascertain what can happen to the individual, whether there be immediate effects or long-term repercussions. But because we want the best of everything and will accept nothing less, the doctor and the practice of medicine in general often becomes the scapegoat.

Rarely do we question our own accountability regarding how we got sick and in the position of needing exotic lifesaving health care in the first place. How many of us breeze through life either ignorant or deceptive about how we abuse ourselves?

Alarmed by a health crisis, we seek miracle cures. Our desperation for an immediate solution fuels a crisis-oriented health care system too concerned with treating symptoms rather than correcting causes.

TREATING SYMPTOMS VERSUS CORRECTING CAUSES

Symptoms are often the last stage of a disease. They are the external warning signs manifested by an internal problem which is often the actual cause of an illness.

Society places too much emphasis on treating our symptoms and nowhere near enough on correcting causes. This practice feeds on itself with seriously increasing consequences—namely, rising costs and a society dependent on crisis health care (Nieman 20)[3].

Ironically, it is more profitable to treat symptoms than to correct causes. In this respect, modern medicine functions the same as it did centuries ago. Returning symptoms mean returning patients. Ignorance on the part of the consumer perpetuates this state of affairs even further by allowing advertisers to lure them with quick-fix remedies. Consequently, we have become a-pill-for-every-problem society. Furthermore, this common acceptance and dependency on drugs contributes to their abuse.

EDUCATION AND PREVENTION

The truth about health combines common sense and knowledge in a program of disease prevention. In this way we rely on ourselves for health maintenance and on doctors for guidance and education instead of crisis care. The undeniable trend of the 1980's is that we are moving away from institutionalized care (the traditional doctor-hospital system) and moving towards self-care (Naisbitt 134). Economics and information are the driving forces.

Awareness of health care issues is fast becoming part of the public consciousness. Health is in our hands—yours and mine. It demands our personal accountability. No longer can we drop our health problems in another's lap. This phenomenon is forever changing the relationship between doctors and patients.

COMMUNICATING WITH DOCTORS

When people possess little knowledge about the workings of their body, they find it difficult to understand doctors and communicate with them. Ignorance puts one at a disadvantage. Having little knowledge about health also results in a lack of accountability. It fosters the practice of dependency on the doctor and crisis care. We tend to believe that it's the doctor's job to ensure our health. Realize, however, that doctors are not responsible for our health.

The doctor must perceive our level of medical knowledge, then explain what our condition is, hopefully in terms we can quickly understand. Without any frame of reference about our bodies, the information doctors provide often fails to integrate into our lives. We have nothing to relate it to. It never registers. This predicament is a vicious cycle, and we are the ultimate losers.

The word *doctor* derives from a Greek word meaning "teacher." Teaching us how to take specific care of ourselves is the greatest service doctors can provide. Medical terminology is the basis of how doctors communicate. Effectively understanding them requires us to learn some rudimentary medical terms* and acquire a basic understanding of how one's body works.

Exactly how does one begin to take care of his or her own health? In the 400 years since the time of Vesalius, much has been learned concerning human anatomy and physiology. In the process it has become clear that certain systems and structures of the body, because of the nature of the tasks they perform, are most important. Therefore, their care and maintenance ensures their efficient functioning, which in turn preserves the health of the body.

* A glossary of basic medical terminology is provided at the back of this book.

DISCOVERING THE TRUTH

In discussing the various components of a healthy lifestyle, however, we tend to neglect a very important aspect of human anatomy involved in the function of the body. Its lack of proper care has become epidemic in our society, resulting in widespread physical and financial distress. Let us explore what this is and why.

3

WHY THE SPINE

"Men occasionally stumble
over the truth,
but most of them pick
themselves up and hurry off
as if nothing had happened."

Sir Winston Churchill

People want to be healthy. But they also want the maintenance of health to take the least amount of time, sacrifice, and money. They would prefer not to give up their habits or be inconvenienced. Human nature naturally looks for the easy way.

Luckily for us, our bodies are designed in such a way that by taking care of one part, that part provides the fundamental basis of good health. What part is that? Your spine. Through the brain and spinal cord the inborn controlling and healing force of your body is at work. The evidence is overwhelming. It's time we examine it.

For too long, health care has been regarded as extremely complex. The truth is, it's quite simple. Health care comes down to taking care of what matters most first, then going from there. Let us piece together why the brain, spinal cord, and spinal column are the most important parts of your body, how they work on a daily basis, and what you can do to care for them, easily, effectively, and permanently.

The brain and spinal cord are the first organs formed after conception. The brain controls the functions of the body by sending and receiving messages through the spinal cord, which extends from the brain. The brain and spinal cord are thus the essential parts of the nervous system, the body's communication network. Without this system, we could not exist.

The brain and spinal cord are the only organs encased in solid bone. Because of their importance, they receive the most protection. The brain is protected by the skull, while the extremely fragile spinal cord is protected by the spinal column. The spinal column is made up of a stack of twenty-four moveable bones called vertebrae. Like a donut, each vertebra has a hollow opening through which the spinal cord passes.

The base of the spinal column is called the sacrum, which comes from ancient Greek and Latin and means "mighty or sacred bone." Made up of five vertebrae that fuse together during childhood, it is the largest bone of the spine. It carries the weight of the upper half of the body and then divides it into the two iliae (hip bones) which transfer the weight to each femur or leg (Figure 3-1).

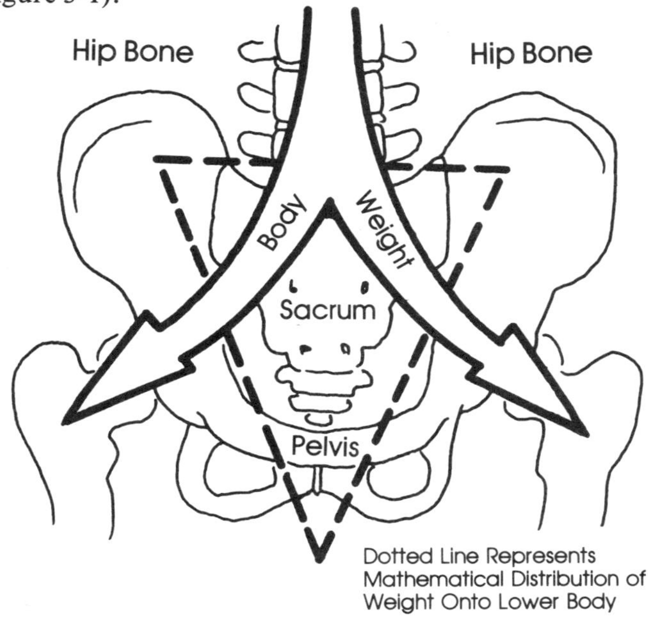

Distribution of Body Weight at Sacrum

Figure 3-1

Adapted from Kapanji, 1974

Below the sacrum lies the coccyx or tail bone, formed by the fusion of four vertebrae. Though the coccyx is not used in supporting the body, it does provide attachment for the gluteus maximus, the large muscle of the buttocks.

The alignment of these vertebrae with respect to each other is of critical importance. Thirty-one pairs of spinal nerves exit the spinal column between each pair of vertebrae and the sacrum and coccyx to reach the various parts of the body. There is only enough space between every two vertebrae for each cluster of nerves to exit. Incorrect alignment of the vertebrae can cause damage to the nerves as they exit the spinal column by impeding the flow of nerve impulses (Rowe 25 ff.).[4]

Most body motion originates at the spinal column (spine). The body's whole physical structure is built upon it. The spine is the body's main source of support, the foundation of your skeletal and muscular structures.

Much like a shock absorber, the spine continually absorbs the physical forces you encounter everyday. Furthermore, the spine is where most of us carry stress.

Together as the body's master control system, the brain, spinal cord, and spinal column are ultimately responsible for controlling and coordinating all systems of the body. Fortunately, this complex communications system is both easy to understand and maintain. Caring for your spine is the basis for taking care of your physical health. Your spine is your lifeline. For further evidence, let's look at how life itself begins.

THE DEVELOPMENT OF HUMAN LIFE

A new life begins when a sperm and egg unite. Soon they develop into a small mass of cells called a blastocyst. By the sixteenth day, a little line resembling an eyelash, called the primitive streak, appears. This is the beginning of the brain and spinal cord, the first tools simultaneously created by our inborn intelligence to facilitate the expression of human potential (Figure 3-2). Human life develops from above down, inside out, that is, from the brain down through the spinal cord and then out through the development of organs and limbs.

The brain is the body's base of operations, the master control center. Everything else—internal organs, bones, muscles—follows the brain in development, as well as being controlled by it.

The spinal cord develops in order to connect the brain with the rest of the growing embryo. Information and instructions pass to and from the brain to the body through the spinal cord. In an adult, the spinal cord terminates at a point slightly above waist level. Here it becomes a series of parallel nerve fibers running downward and out of the vertebrae of the lower spine. These strands resemble a horse's tail and thus are known as the *cauda equina* (Latin for "horse's tail").

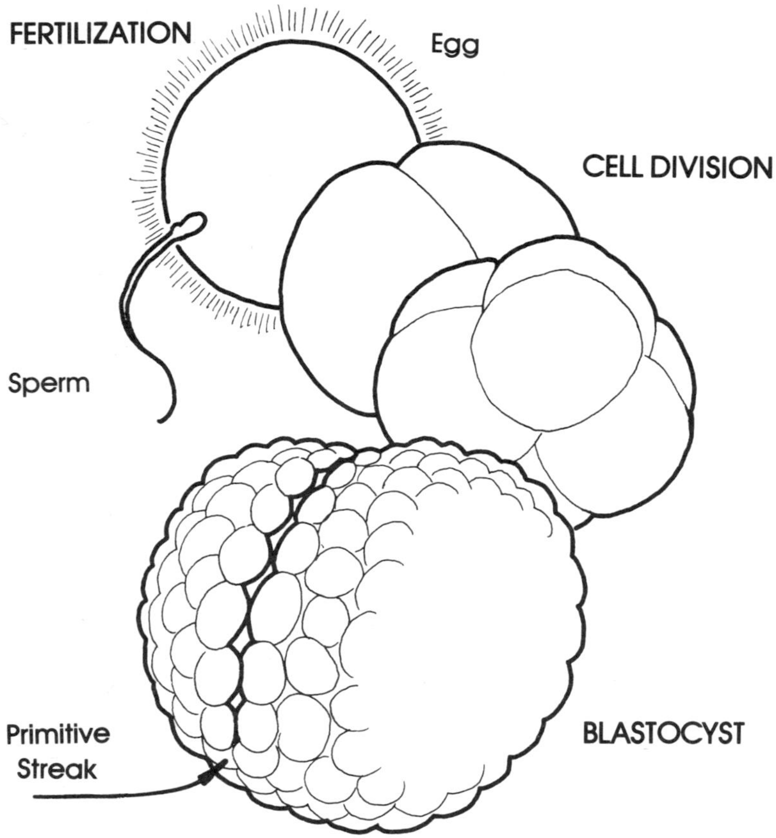

Figure 3-2 EARLY HUMAN DEVELOPMENT

The peripheral nervous system forms as nerves branch out from the spinal cord and cranium to reach each of the billions of cells in the body. This vast and intricate network coordinates every function of the body.

Afferent nerves are that portion of the nerve branches that

are receptors of sensory stimuli from all parts of the body. The information they receive is sent to the brain through the spinal cord. There the brain processes the information and formulates a response. Other nerve branches, called efferent nerves, carry the brain's message back to the appropriate part or parts of the body for implementation.

As the fetus continues its development, the spine takes on a shape called the epicyclic arc, which is a curve from the back of the head through the rest of the spine. This arc is the structural basis for physical development of the body after birth. After spending nine months floating in the womb, a newborn must be prepared for a major factor of life: gravity (Figure 3-3).

Gravity greatly affects the spine. A newborn must develop the strength and leverage to hold itself upright against this force. Immediately after birth, the body begins developing this capacity. The shape of the spine changes as additional spinal curvature begins to develop.

The strength of any curve or structure can be expressed in terms of engineering properties. If you find the number of curves an object has, square it and add one, the result equals the relative resilience and mobility of the curve. The spine of a newborn has one long curve: One squared plus one equals two. The relative strength factor is quite low. This is why a newborn has little control over the movement of its head.

Between two and four months of an infant's age, the neck curve begins to develop. This curve gives the baby the strength and leverage necessary to control the movement of its head. Thus, the main curve has taken a segment of itself and created an additional smaller curve, called the cervical curve (Figure 3-4).

Leverage in the spine can be expressed in terms of the size or mass of the body being moved versus the length of a particular spinal segment it uses as foundation. In order to gain more leverage, the body has begun to transform the original, long curve into smaller sections.

At this stage of the baby's development, there are three curves: The curve starting at the back of the head (the occipital curve), the curve of the neck (the cervical curve), and the curve that goes down the rest of the spine, (the remainder of the epicyclic arc). The strength factor now increases from two (one squared plus one) to ten (three squared plus one).

As arm and leg muscles develop, the baby learns to assume an upright posture and a fourth curve forms. Located in the lower back, it is the lumbar curve (Figure 3-5).

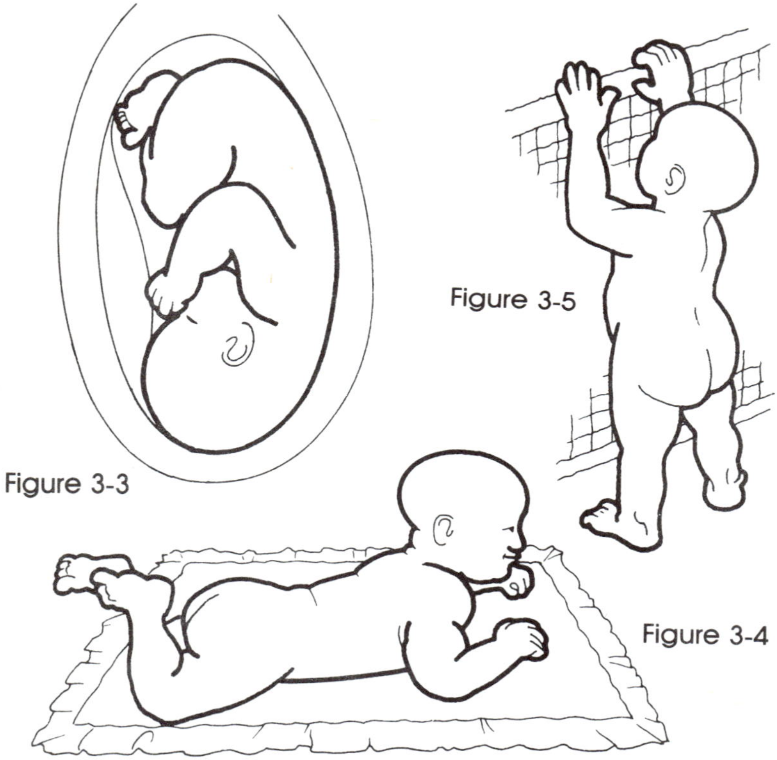

DEVELOPMENT OF SPINAL CURVATURE

The fifth curve, the pelvic curve, extends from the lower back into the sacrum and down into the coccyx, commonly known as the tailbone. This provides a strength factor of five squared plus one, or twenty-six (Pettibon *Spinal Angles* 44).[5]

In a matter of nine to fifteen months, then, the baby has gone from a strength factor of two to a strength factor of twenty-six.

Physical coordination advances steadily. All of the muscles are now working against a proper set of spinal curves, ideally leveraged for strength, flexibility, and control (Figure 3-6).

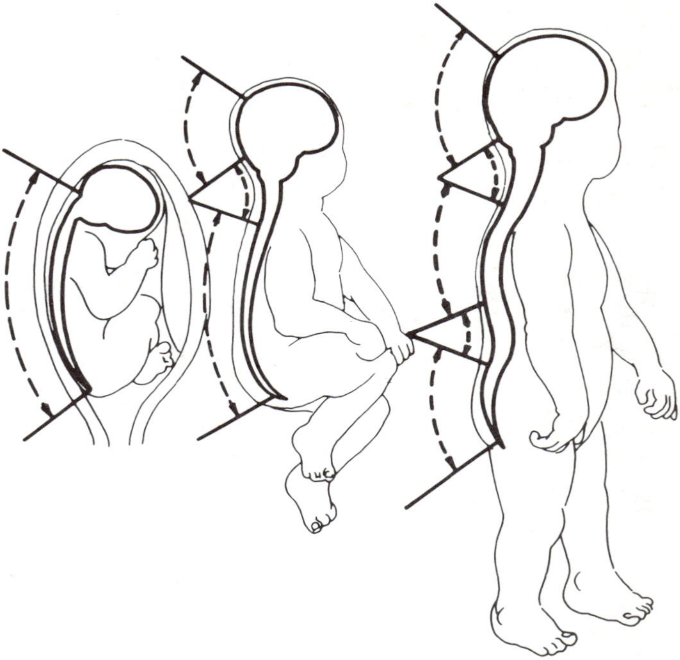

STRENGTH FACTORS OF SPINAL CURVATURE DEVELOPMENT

Figure 3-6 Adapted from Pettibon, 1979

The child is able to move about and function in ways it never could before. The coordination of other muscles can now take effect. After the child learns to walk and run, it moves on to more sophisticated and controlled actions with its arms and legs. Further development increases and refines flexibility, motion, coordination, and strength.

Clearly, one can see the importance of the spine in the early development of every human being.

4

YOUR SPINE IS A SUPERSTRUCTURE

THE SPINE IS IN BACK OF THE BODY
BUT SHOULD BE KEPT
IN THE FRONT OF THE MIND

One can easily see that the spine must be in good working order for the body to be likewise. The health of the body is greatly influenced by the position and condition of the spinal column and the functional capability of the nervous system.[6] This is a fundamental concept of *The Real Truth About Health*.

Understanding the spine is not as complicated as the work it performs. The spine is built like a bridge. It can be reduced to lines and numbers. A little simple math, two or three terms to learn, a few concepts to grasp, and you're on your way.

The twenty-four individual segments, called vertebrae, which compose the spine are grouped into three primary sections. Together the three sections act as a unit, the result being the coordinated and controlled movement of the body.

The top section, known as the cervical spine, contains the first seven vertebrae. The skull itself sits on the first vertebra, called the atlas. The six vertebrae below form the neck.

The middle section is called the thoracic region. It contains twelve vertebrae, each with a rib attached.

The bottom section, known as the lumbar spine, contains the last five vertebrae, which sit upon the sacrum and coccyx.

A normal spine, when viewed from the front, is perfectly straight. It follows the physical center of a person's body (Figure 4-1). Viewed from the side, the normal spine is a series of graceful, undulating curves of specific dimensions and diameters (Pettibon *Theory* 36 ff.), (Figure 4-2).

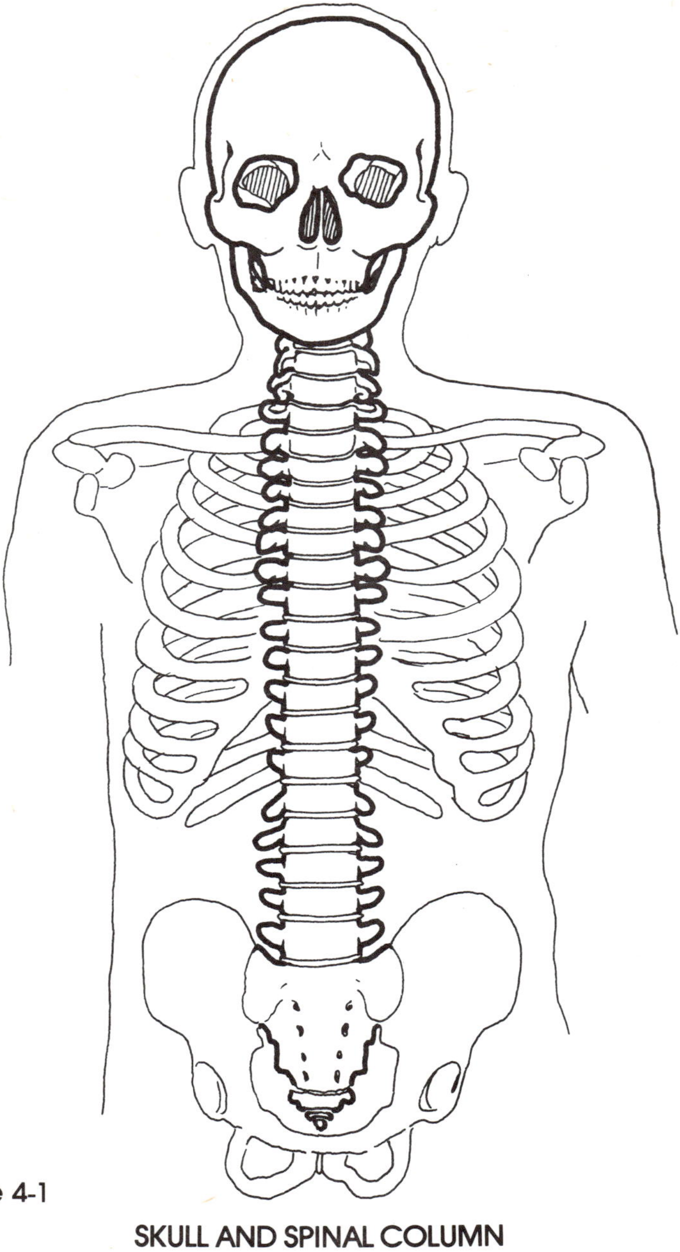

Figure 4-1

SKULL AND SPINAL COLUMN

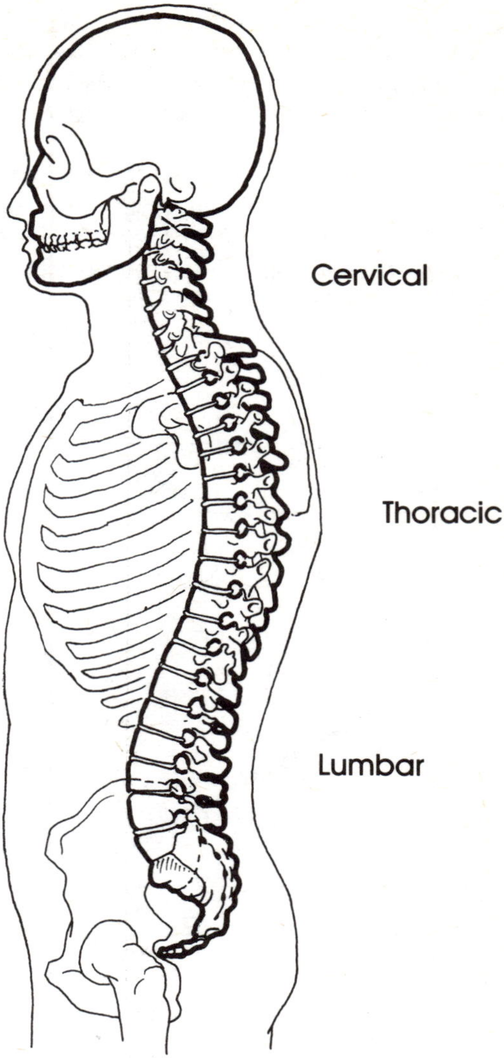

Figure 4-2

SKULL AND SPINAL COLUMN, SIDE VIEW

SPINAL CURVES AND CURVATURE

The curves in the spine enable the muscles in those areas to function optimally. Each curve blends perfectly into the one above and below it. Ideally, the curves are of specific diameters.

In a normal spine, the height of the curve is equal to the radius of the curve (Pettibon *Spinal Angles* 44). This describes the extent of the curve present to give the optimum blend of strength and control of body movement. The amount of curvature dictates the amount of motion possible from that area of the spine (Figure 4-3).

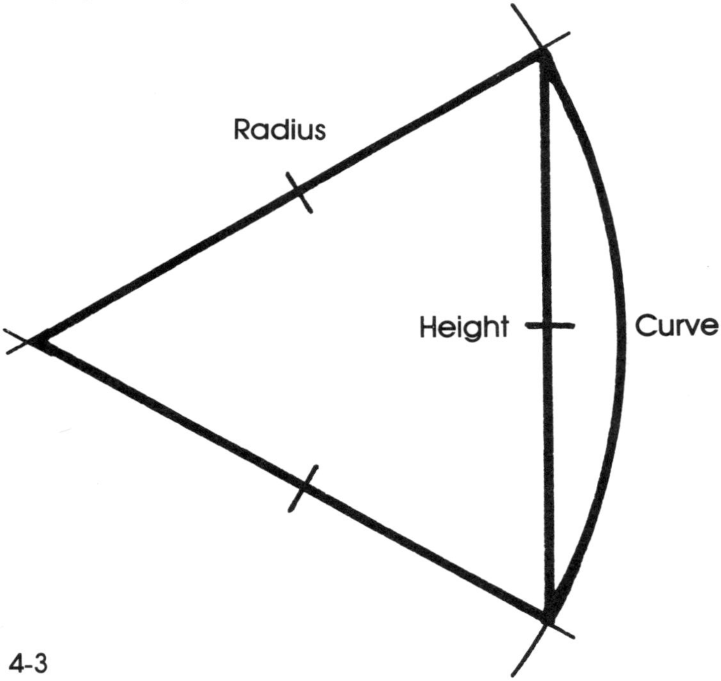

Figure 4-3

HEIGHT OF CURVE EQUALS ITS RADIUS

A healthy spinal column means a proper balance of the curves, that is, not having too much or too little curvature. Curvature provides the strength and leverage for the body to have motion. A frequent problem arises from having too little curvature, which causes increased resistance against the muscles. The result is that the energy expended by the muscle is less effective in producing motion because it results in increased muscle use throughout the entire range of motion. Ultimately, the muscle suffers fatigue (Imrie 53).

Too much curvature, on the other hand, causes the vertebrae to be moved out of place and overly forced into the curves. This can compress the spine too much and result in shortening and tightening of the muscles. Over a period of time the muscles begin to lose their normal elasticity (Root 119).

Without proper spinal curvature, movement of the body is difficult, and the ability to resist force and stress is greatly diminished because leverage has been lost.

SPINAL LIGAMENTS AND MUSCLES

Ligaments are tough, elastic tissue that connect bones to other bone and serve as reinforcement for joints. The spinal column is covered by two main ligaments that run the length of it, the anterior and posterior longitudinal ligaments. Also supporting the spinal column are smaller ligaments that provide stabilization and direct the motion of individual vertebra.

Muscles are contractible fibers that respond to nerve impuses. Four primary muscle groups help support the spinal column and provide movement of the body. In the front, the spine is supported by the abdominal muscles and in the back by the extensor muscles. Lateral muscles give support and motion to the sides of the spine. Hip muscles coordinate the relationship of the spinal column to the lower extremities.

With the spine providing a stable foundation, the larger muscles of the back have the necessary leverage to move the body. This foundation allows stabilization at the fulcrum, or point of greatest stress. The back muscles not only stabilize the body but also provide a counter balance to external forces. Opposing resistance develops through the use of more than one muscle. Anywhere there is motion by the body, there is also a carefully orchestrated set of mutually opposing muscles.

We are fortunate that we don't have to think about muscle

movement while dealing with a force or a load. Always keeping us balanced is an innate function of the body. The way in which the body's weight is carried is another miracle of the engineering of the human frame.

In fact, your body is marvelously arranged and organized (Figure 4-4). If you took two bathroom scales and stood with one foot on each, exactly half your weight should register on each scale. This is an excellent way to tell how your weight is distributed and a good indication of the position of the spinal column itself.

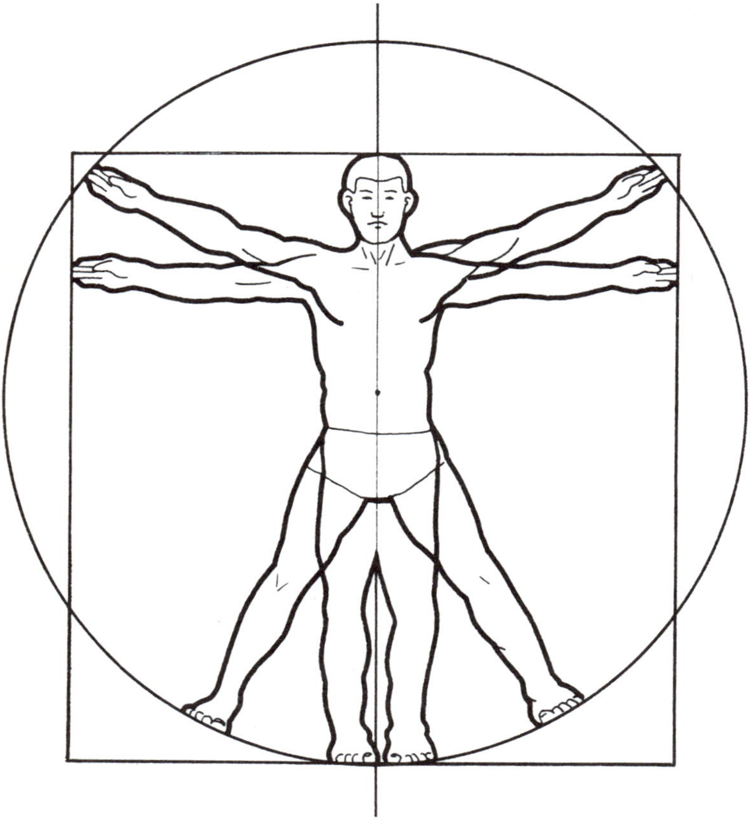

ORGANIZATION OF THE HUMAN BODY

Figure 4-4

Incidentally, balance is an important factor in the engineering of robotics. A robot needs a low center of gravity to counter the weight held away from the center of gravity, so that leverage is still maintained. In people, the vertical axis, (the up and down center line) runs through the skull, the center of the body, and down between the legs, knees, and ankles.

An important part of health, from a structural perspective, is the importance of the body balancing its weight equally on both sides. When more weight is carried on one side than the other, that side of the body is under greater stress and subjected to more wear. Over a period of time that side of the body begins to deteriorate. Joints are literally worn out from stress. The result is similar to the front end of a car being out of alignment and causing abnormal wear on the tires.

For such an important organ, the spinal cord is amazingly delicate. If you took the spinal cord out of the spinal column and rolled it between your fingers, it would turn to paste. This is why spinal injuries occur so frequently and are so dangerous.

When the spinal column is out of alignment, normal nerve function is impaired. When nerves don't work correctly, messages to and from the various parts of the body are not properly conveyed. Either the brain cannot properly communicate with a particular part of the body, or that part of the body cannot respond properly to the brain or both. Although that part may be in good condition, it won't work correctly unless the brain can communicate with it.

DESIGN AND FUNCTION OF INDIVIDUAL VERTEBRA

Now that we have discussed the spine as a wholly functioning unit, let's look at the units of vertebrae of which it is made. The word vertebra comes from the Latin *vetere* meaning "to turn." The properties inherent in each vertebra allow the spine to perform its many tasks.

Each vertebra is composed of two primary portions, front and back, differentiated by function and structure. The front half of the vertebra, called the body section, is a massive cylinder of bone whose primary function is to bear weight. In other words, it holds us upright. This front part of each spinal vertebra is uniquely designed to absorb forces the body encounters. The inside of the front portion of each vertebra is honeycombed, one of the strongest structural configurations known, providing maximum strength with minimum weight.

The back half of the vertebra is composed of the neural arch, with three projections. Some of the projections serve as attachments for muscles. Others serve as joints to produce guidance for motion with adjacent vertebrae. Depending on the motion required, part of the spine becomes rigid as a supportive structure for the motion that takes place above or below it (Figure 4-5).

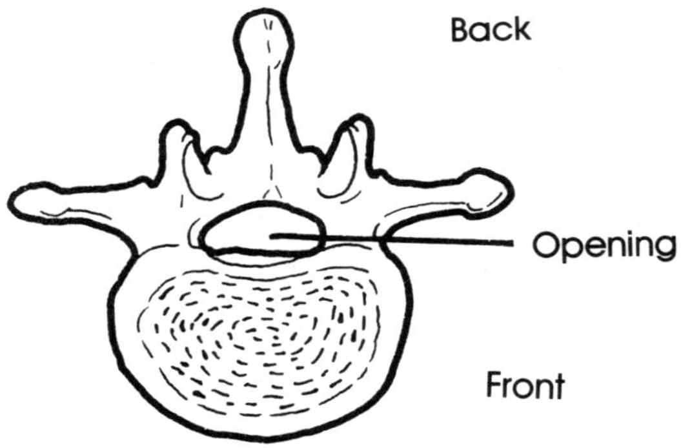

TOP VIEW OF VERTEBRA

Figure 4-5

The hollow opening within each vertebra houses and protects the spinal cord. Think of the vertebrae as forming a tunnel through which the spinal cord passes.

Between each two vertebrae is an opening through which a cluster of nerves branch out from the spinal cord. These nerves connect the spinal cord and brain to every cell and organ in the body.

Each pair of vertebrae come together to form a facet joint. On the front half of the facet joint, the back portions of the massive cylinder of bone and the back portions of the disc form the front half of the neural foramina. On the back, the extension of the pedicle down to the facet joint and the opposing portion of the joint below form the back portion of the neural foramina. This creates a little opening called the intervertebral foramina through which the nerves exit the spinal cord and extend to all parts of the body (Figure 4-6).

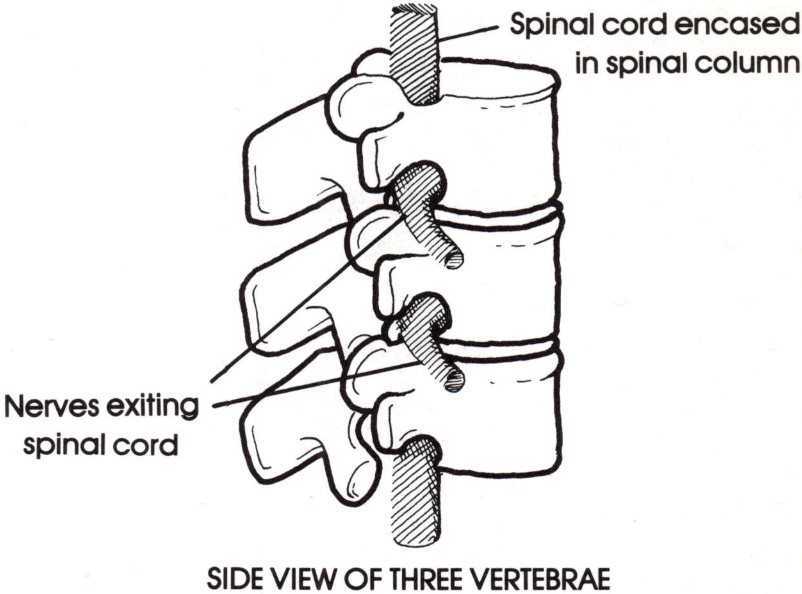

Figure 4-6

In effect, intervertebral foramina are formed by the exact position of individual vertebra. There is only enough space to allow the cluster of nerves to pass through (Leach 51).[7] This offers the delicate spinal cord the greatest amount of protection. This also means however, that maintaining the correct position of the spinal column is essential.

When the vertebrae are out of alignment, the opening they form for the nerve cluster to pass through is reduced. What is commonly known as a "pinched nerve" may result. The flow of nerve impulses is impeded, thereby disrupting the operation of the nervous system itself (Leach 49 ff.),[8] (Figure 4-7).

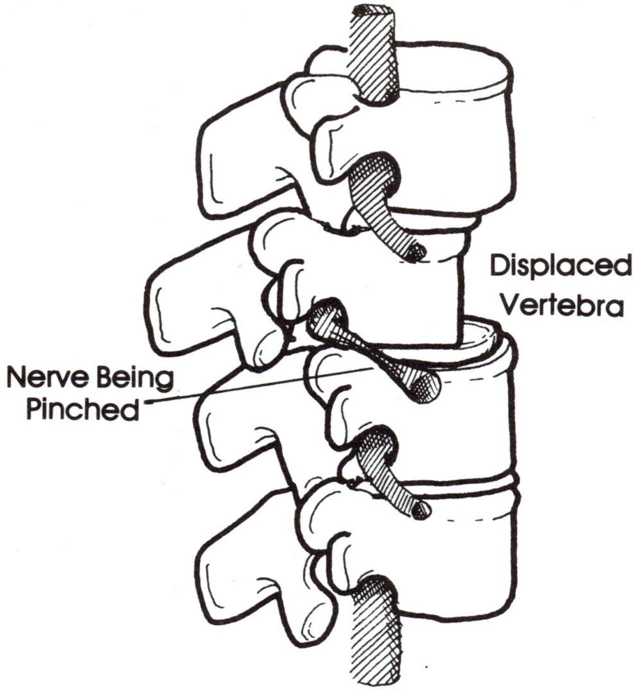

PINCHED NERVE

Figure 4-7

CONSTRUCTION AND FUNCTION OF DISCS

Intervertebral discs which separate the vertebrae act as shock absorbers and allow motion to take place within the spinal column. Discs work like ball bearings, enabling the vertebrae to rock back and forth and pivot. This motion occurs in the disc center, known as the nucleus pulposus.

Similiar to the construction of an automobile tire, discs contain layers running in different directions, thus providing added strength. The outer part of each disc consists of a cartilage-like fiber called the annulus fibrosus. The internal portion is a gelatinous mass of protein called collagen. As a tire's pressure results from being filled with compressed air, a disc's pressure comes from its high water content (approximately 80%).

The nucleus of the disc distributes pressure in all directions, enabling the joint to bear considerable weight and absorb jolts to the spine.

The health of the discs is ensured by the friction and heat caused by motion of the spine (Pettibon *Theory* 62). In this manner, the discs are nourished and relieved of their waste products. Therefore, the spine's capability of a full range of motion is dependent on the health of the discs. And the health of the discs is dependent on regular motion of the spinal column. Also, the position of the spinal vertebrae, if abnormal, can cause stress and physical damage to the discs by improperly distributing forces and weight (Figure 4-8).

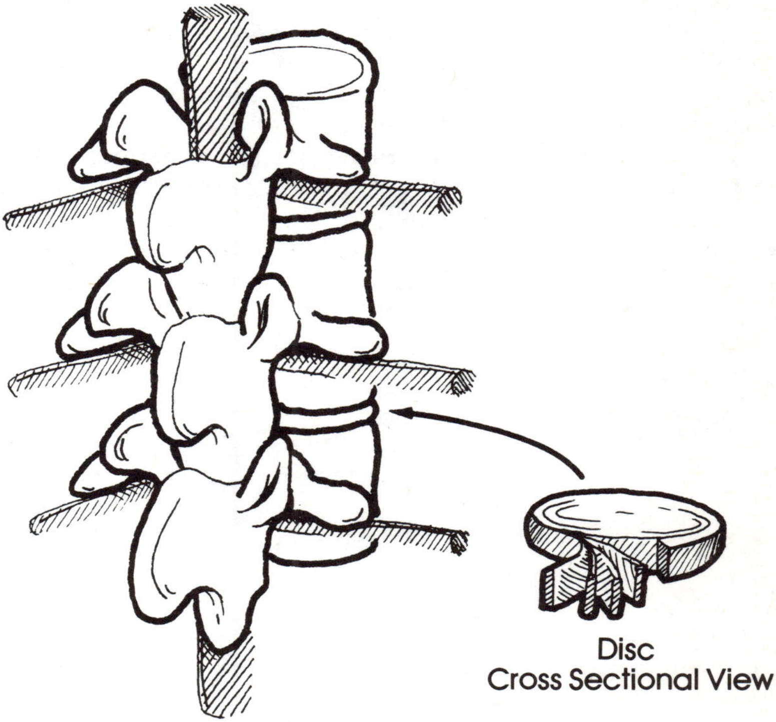

REAR VIEW OF THE THORACIC SPINE

Figure 4-8

THE OCCIPUT, ATLAS, AND AXIS

The only spinal vertebrae that don't have discs are the atlas and the axis. The occiput, the bottom part of the skull, is where the weight of the skull rests on top of the atlas vertebra, which is the top vertebra of the spinal column.

The atlas is named after the mythical Greek god Atlas, who supported the world on his shoulders. The atlas vertebra, positioned properly under the skull, ensures that the skull is perfectly balanced on top of the cervical spine. The rocking of the skull on the atlas allows for up and down motion of the head, as when nodding.

The axis is the vertebra immediately below the atlas, supporting both the atlas and skull. The axis contains the odontoid process, a post-like projection located at the front of the axis which fits into the opening of the atlas above it. Turning the head from side to side, as in gesturing "No," turns the atlas around the odontoid process of the axis (Figure 4-9).

Sometimes injuries or problems of the spine necessitate a trip to the doctor. There are a variety of doctors whose practice include the study and treatment of the spine. Of them, chiropractors are highly specialized, treating disorders of the spine almost exclusively. Their profession is a story in itself.

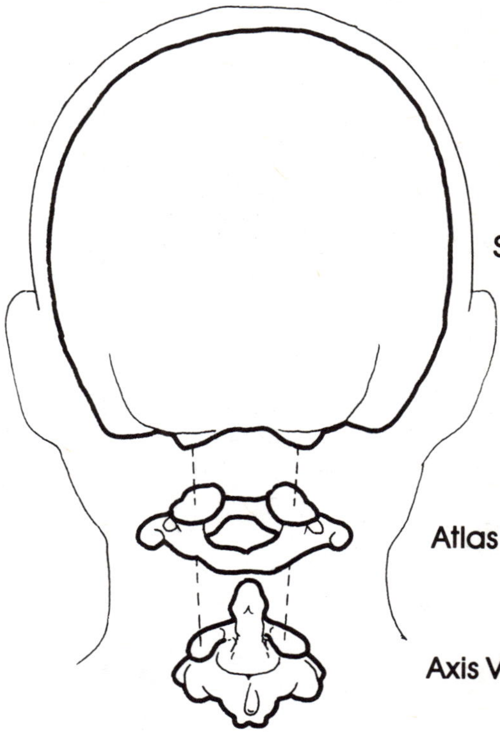

SKULL, ATLAS, AND AXIS VERTEBRAE

Figure 4-9

5

CHIROPRACTIC: THE HEALTH CARE ENIGMA

"There is a principle which is a bar
against all information, which is
proof against all argument and which
cannot fail to keep a man in
everlasting ignorance. That principle is,
'Condemnation before investigation.' "

Herbert Spencer

Chiropractic and chiropractors are like the spine itself: often misunderstood and overlooked. A profession that claims to be the world's largest natural healing art, however, shouldn't be taken lightly (Leach 26). Upwards of ten million people a year seek chiropractic services, a fact which indicates the epidemic of back problems in this country. According to one estimate, one-fourth of the population of the United States has been to a chiropractor at one time or another (Leach 6).

Back disabilities account for a substantial number of insurance claims. Twenty percent of all Workers' Compensation claims are for back injuries (Rowe 6).[9] Yet the public has little accurate knowledge about chiropractors or what they do. Fewer still know what chiropractic is. Chiropractic's story began with a discovery on September 18, 1895, by Daniel David Palmer, known to his contemporaries as "D.D." Palmer's discovery was a new method of health care, the culmination of years of study in many different fields.

Palmer's contribution to health care was the systematic arranging of the philosophy, science, and art of chiropractic. His contemplative nature served to create the philosophy of the new healing art. His self-taught background in anatomy and physiology provided him with the necessary scientific fundamentals. His willingness to take action and experiment resulted in the very first chiropractic adjustment.

D.D. was born on March 7, 1845, near Toronto, Canada, one of six children born to Thomas and Catherine Palmer. His father was a shoemaker and later a grocer. D.D. and his brother, Thomas J., were taught by a country schoolmaster, one John Black, who gave them a basic education, including instruction in natural sciences and classical languages.

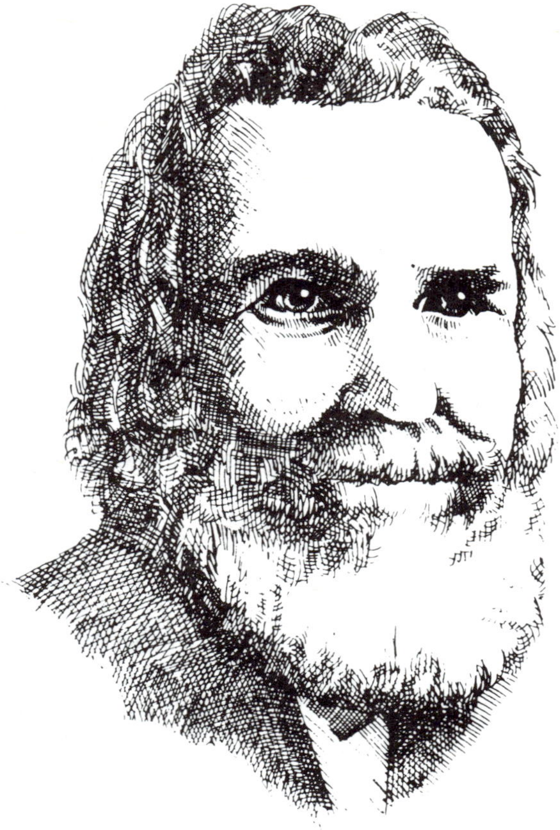

D. D. PALMER

During the Civil War, many Americans fled to Canada in order to avoid the combat. This swelled the Canadian labor pool, so Palmer sought employment in the United States. He and his brother arrived in 1865. D.D. was twenty. Eight months after his arrival, he became a schoolmaster in Muscatine County, Iowa. He taught fifty pupils in the classic one-room schoolhouse of the prairies.

Educators of the era were partial to mottos and simple poems designed to indoctrinate youth with a proper moral foundation. D.D. was no exception. Here are a few of his own thoughts, testimony to his life-long concern for a healthy physical and spiritual life:

> Excelsior, higher and higher, but only step by step.
> Study first, play afterwards.
> The best physicians are Dr. Diet,
> Dr. Quiet, and Dr. Merryman.
> The mill cannot grind with the water that is past.
> Little deeds are like little seeds,
> they grow to flowers, or to weeds.
> He who obeys God's laws finds him a father. He who disobeys them, finds him a judge [Gielow 10].[10]

After working as a teacher for several years, Palmer bought property and began raising bees and fruit trees. Later he added a nursery operation. When John Mason's invention of the canning jar in 1857 made preserving foodstuffs possible, Palmer capitalized on it, spending the better part of ten years selling berries and honey.

Palmer was also a very religious man. He read his Bible frequently, underlining lines and verses to such an extent that the entire book was black with markings.

In 1881, Palmer moved with his wife Louvenia to the city of What Cheer, Iowa, where he operated a grocery store. There his third child, Bartlett Joshua, or B.J., was born on September 14, 1882.

Through fervent lifelong reading and study habits, Palmer nurtured his interest in science and the development of humanity. There was an insistent whisper in the ear of this man who had not yet found his proper niche in life. D.D.'s style was to move onward and upward, hoping to find opportunities to increase his knowledge and utilize his talents.

Such an opportunity was provided by a man named Paul Caster, who was gaining recognition as an outstanding healer in Ottumwa, Iowa. He had an extremely large practice as a magnetic healer, a healing art introduced to the United States in the 1830s.

The origins of magnetic healing date back to the time of Paracelsus, a Swiss physician who lived from 1493 to 1541. Paracelsus believed all matter, organic and inorganic, was endowed with its own spirit. According to him, each person possessed magnetic powers capable of attracting both good and evil. He taught that a magnetic field exuded from human beings, that it could be guided by their wills, influencing the minds and bodies of others. It was Paracelsus' opinion that "A physician should be the servant of nature, not her enemy. He should be able to guide and direct her in her struggle for life, and not throw, by his unreasonable influence, fresh obstacles in the way of recovery" (Gielow 35).

Paracelsus' concepts surfaced again two centuries later through the work of Franz Anton Mesmer, born in Austria in 1734. Mesmer treated patients using magnetic power, passing his hands over their bodies as a healing treatment.

Palmer lived at a time of experimentation in all areas of health care. His quest for knowledge prompted him to read the scientific volumes of the period. There was latitude for investigation in many directions, with few regulations of any kind. Phrenology, naturopathy, allopathy, eclectic medicine, homeopathy, physical therapeutics, and osteopathy were present or on the horizon of consideration by the health-conscious and those dedicated to the improvement of humanity. Expansion was the vogue of the 19th century. The nation was maturing. The soil of intellectual pursuit was fertile. Many seeds were planted and encouraged to grow.

Palmer found the philosophical concepts of magnetic healing very attractive. He visited Paul Caster to learn more about magnetic healing firsthand. After further study on his own, Palmer began his own practice in Burlington, Iowa, along the banks of the Mississippi in 1886. He later moved to Davenport, Iowa, in 1887.

Within a couple of years, Palmer developed a steady clientele. He also set in motion a very effective advertising program, selling himself through the *Educator*, Palmer's own newsletter which he sent to patients and the general public.

Palmer, now forty-three with a growing practice, leased additional space in 1888. Much of Palmer's magnetic healing practice was based on a book titled *Vital Magnetism, the Life Fountain*. The author was E.D. Babbit, D.M. According to Babbit's book, magnetic healing called for precise hand movements by the practitioner, who had to prepare himself mentally and physically to be effective. Babbit wrote about the importance of maintaining high personal integrity as well as a high level of physical and spiritual health on the part of the practitioner. He stressed the importance of a diet consisting of fresh fruits and vegetables and refraining from drugs and alcohol. He also advocated daily meditation and self-examination.

Notes from Palmer's journal indicate his own thoughts about magnetic healing:

> Commence treatment by allaying the fear of disease or drugs.
> Silently measure the patient.
> Grief causes suffering & disease.
> Give yourself a treatment, first be sure that you are O.K.
> The mind must be cured as well as the body, as the mind so is the body [Gielow 56].

Over the next several years, Palmer's practice blossomed. He treated many patients, and though there were skeptics of his work, he had a positive relationship with the community.

Palmer avidly continued reading books, newspapers, and periodicals. He observed and carefully scrutinized all forms of health practice. Palmer had a unique need to study. He lived with two intellectual sides, the scientific and the metaphysical. Eventually, the pragmatic and the abstract sides were to meld in the creation of a well-defined and dramatically different healing art, that of chiropractic.

Harvey Lillard, a janitor in the building where Palmer practiced magnetic healing, was under Palmer's care and proved to be a perplexing case. He had been nearly deaf for many years. Palmer had treated him by a series of magnetic healing passes over his spine. In doing so, he had noticed a peculiar bump on the man's back. When he rubbed this area, he determined there was something out of place.

Palmer tried to reduce the bump over a period of time. As his various approaches failed, he became more aggressive in his attempts, using his hands to push on the man's spine. Ultimately the bump, a vertebra, slipped back into place, resulting in an improvement in the man's hearing within a short period of time.

Once Palmer recognized that vertebrae could move out of place, disrupt the normal flow of nerve impulses and impair health, his objective was to develop a reliable method of restoring their position. Palmer was already known as a talented man at bone setting. He was aware of the exact relationships between bone structures. His first spinal adjustment lacked the specific calculations now employed by many chiropractors, but its effect was the same: to reposition vertebrae so that the segments of the spine are in proper anatomical proximity to those above and below. In his book *The Science, Art and Philosophy of Chiropractic,* D.D. Palmer wrote of his discovery:

> Shortly after this relief from deafness, I had a patient with a case of heart trouble that was not improving. I examined the spine and found a displaced vertebra pressing against the nerves which innervate the heart. I adjusted the vertebra and gave immediate relief—nothing 'accidental' or 'crude' about this.
>
> Then I began to reason if two diseases, so dissimiliar as deafness and heart trouble, came from impingement, a pressure on nerves, were not other diseases due to a similar cause? Thus the science (knowledge) and art (adjusting) of Chiropractic were formed at that time [52].

With the conviction of having made a profound inroad into the mysteries of the potential causes of disease, Palmer became quite reclusive. All experimentation was done in private. Heavy drapes darkened his work room windows. He allowed no one to observe his palpatings (examinations performed with the hands and fingers) and spinal adjustments.

Palmer had good reason for being cautious. He was afraid of having his ideas and methodology stolen. He was also concerned about repercussions from the medical profession. At that time, doctors were afraid of the potentially adverse affects of twisting or moving the neck in any way. Since severe criticism could cause him ruin, Palmer protected himself with secrecy.

The practice of moving spinal bones was not new, however, having originated with the ancient Egyptians and Chinese.

Walking on the backs of the very ill was a common treatment, though results were mixed. Some got better, while others never got up again. The ancient practitioners didn't know exactly what they were doing. They only knew that somehow the back affected the rest of the body.

It would be centuries later, at the time of Palmer's first spinal adjustment, that the truth was revealed. Palmer knew that he had discovered something of great potential for humanity. Initially though, he was unsure himself of exactly what he was doing and how his methods worked.

Desiring a Greek name for his new health science, Palmer consulted a patient and friend, the Reverend Samuel H. Weed, a scholar of Greek literature. Palmer eventually chose "chiropractic" from the words *cheir*, which means "hand" and *praktos* meaning "done." This new healing art was literally done by skilled use of the hands.

Palmer continued his search into the causes of disease, experimenting with chiropractic adjusting and documenting his thoughts and findings. The 19th century was about to close, with massive changes still to come. Major philosophical shifts in education and science were developing worldwide. There was more scientific exploration in progress than the world had ever known before.

Many innovations of this time originated in Germany, a nation determined to become the leader in all scientific pursuits, including medicine. Palmer would later find these changes aggravating obstacles to the growth of his new profession.

D.D. Palmer was a graduate of the old method of education, that is, to teach a craft without offering education in other backgrounds of knowledge. Most people before 1900 gained their education and began endeavors in their chosen fields through this method. Palmer was no exception.

At first he attempted to start his school teaching only chiropractic. But soon he discovered that teaching a single subject would not suffice because of the changing times. Palmer found it necessary to teach chiropractic with the support of other relevant topics. Students were thus provided with a wider background in anatomy and physiology, particularly regarding the spinal column and nervous system.

In January, 1898, William A. Seeley became Palmer's first full-fledged student. The next candidate was Dr. A.P. Davis, a medical practitioner and an osteopath. The tuition was five hundred dollars and the course lasted nine months (Gielow 91). Initially, Palmer wanted to instruct only two students at a time. From this meager beginning, the educational process was underway at the Palmer School and Infirmary of Chiropractic at the corner of Second and Brady Streets in Davenport, Iowa. The chiropractic school had slow beginnings, graduating only twenty students from 1897 to 1906 (CiRullo 13).[11]

An avid reader and a student of virtually every healing persuasion then known in this country, Palmer was most capable to set forth the premise that chiropractic was separate and distinct from any other health field. As an investigator, he had the strengths of a pragmatist as well as those of an idealist. Palmer wrote in his newsletter *The Chiropractic:*

> We are living in an age of wonders. Every day we are surprised at some new invention, and yet many of these new ideas are so simple and easily understood that we wonder why our grandparents did not know of them.
>
> Today we have a comprehensible explanation of the fundamental principles upon which all these cures are made. Today the causes of disease are being located and those causes corrected just as surely as any mechanic would find the cause of inharmony or wrong-working in a piano, wagon, watch, engine or other machine.
>
> A human being is a human machine, and like a machine, would run smoothly, without any friction, if every part was in its proper place. If every bone, every nerve and all the blood vessels, and muscles, were just right, there would be nothing wrong.
>
> Disease is the effect or result of some part of the body being disarranged. To put them in their proper place would give the diseased person ease and allow nature to rebuild without being obstructed.
>
> If every part of the human body was in its natural place there would be no friction, no inflammation, no fever, no weakness. Why not remove the pressure, adjust the framework, and take the strain off those sensitive nerves [3]?

As to the question of what is chiropractic healing, Palmer wrote in his newsletter:

> It is a scientific method of treating diseases. It is a new and radical departure from all other known methods. Chiropractic healing uses no drugs or chemicals, no surgical operations.
>
> Chiropractic healers need a knowledge of the anatomical construction of the human body and the physiological laws governing the distribution of its vital fluids and forces.
>
> Chiropractic healing simplifies the treatment of the most painful and prostrating forms of disease. The human body is a very sensitive and delicately constructed piece of machinery. There are numerous accidents which are liable to injure and misplace the various parts of this highly sensitive, nervous system. All motor and sensory powers are derived through the nerves. How necessary then is it that they should be perfectly free to act? Strange but true, all the nerves of the body may be reached and acted upon by the hands.
>
> Man is a physical and spiritual epitome of the Universe. The spiritual is the cause of action. Action is life. The spiritual always did exist, always will. It is eternal, it is changeless. The linking together of the spiritual and the physical makes it our duty to keep the corporeal frame in proper alignment [4].

D.D. Palmer is the acknowledged Father of Chiropractic. By 1896, he had coined the words *vertebral subluxation* and *adjustment* (described in detail in chapter seven) to identify his methods exactly. Palmer registered and copyrighted the root word *chiroprac-,* and the suffixes *-tic* and *-tor* used with it (CiRullo 12). There are no such words as chiropractory, chiropractice, or chiropraxy.

On January 6, 1902, four students graduated as Doctors of Chiropractic. Among them was D.D.'s son, Bartlett Joshua, or B.J. as he is often known. Later that year, D.D. Palmer left for the West Coast to lecture and start another school, leaving B.J. more or less in charge of the facility. The school was now called the Palmer School of Chiropractic. D.D., however, returned a couple of years later, as his endeavors on the West Coast met with little success. Together, father and son established an equal partnership that continued until May of 1906.

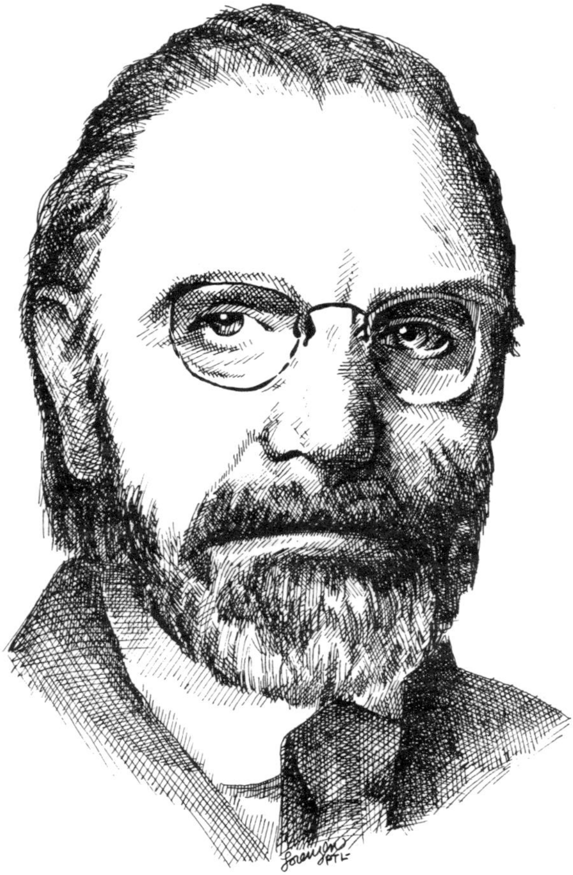

B. J. PALMER

All did not go well between them. There was tension between father and son. Both men were strong-willed and their opinions differed about how to run the school. Many of their problems were caused by the growing pains of chiropractic itself. Likewise, the Palmers had to deal with changes in education and mounting pressure from the medical profession, which by this time had become well organized. Chiropractic was looked upon as serious competition.

Later in 1906, D.D. sold the Palmer School of Chiropractic to B.J., who was rapidly becoming the driving force of the emerging chiropractic profession. D.D. traveled back and forth to the West Coast several times before he died in Los Angeles on October 20, 1913, at age sixty-eight.

In 1910, B.J. had seen demonstrations of the X-ray machine, invented by Dr. William Roentgen in 1895, the same year that chiropractic was founded. B.J., progressively minded, believed X-rays provided an excellent diagnostic tool for chiropractors by providing a visual method to analyze the spinal column. To him, this was the wave of the future.

The contribution of B.J. Palmer to chiropractic was that of its developer. B.J. built the first chiropractic research and development clinic. He also wrote, published, and copyrighted the first book on the science, art, and philosophy of chiropractic. He was responsible for forming the first parent or national chiropractic association and its state associations with twelve other graduates of the Palmer School of Chiropractic. Entitled The Universal Chiropractor's Association, now known as The International Chiropractor's Association, it was the only national chiropractic association in existence until 1921.

The Palmers developed chiropractic as a way to restore and maintain the internal controlling force contained within every person. Though they were acutely aware of external causes of disease such as viruses, they realized the necessity of properly maintaining the function of this inner force. Studying this inborn or innate intelligence became the basis of chiropractic philosophy.

6

INNATE INTELLIGENCE: THE POWER WITHIN YOU

"It is my conviction from having watched a great many babies grow up, that all of humanity is born a genius but then becomes de-geniused very rapidly by unfavorable circumstances and by the frustration of their extraordinary built-in capabilities."

R. Buckminster Fuller

Much of chiropractic's evolution was due to the efforts of B.J. Palmer. This man authored and published over forty books, along with countless brochures, pamphlets, and articles on the subject of chiropractic and health care delivery. B.J. was an international traveler who developed one of the world's finest osteological collections. He had great oratory skills as well as accomplished musical talents. B.J. was also a pioneer in other fields such as radio and television. He owned the first radio station west of the Mississippi. One of his employees, Ronald Reagan, would go on to become President of the United States.

Establishing chiropractic as a legitimate health care system was one of B.J. Palmer's priorities. He led the fight to have chiropractic included in state and federal licensing laws. Kansas was the first state to grant a license to practice chiropractic in 1914. Louisiana was the last in 1973. The federal government did not recognize chiropractic until the Medicare law was passed in 1972.

B.J. Palmer taught chiropractic to thousands of students. He took this infant profession and developed it into the largest natural healing art in the world. He obviously lived a full and productive life, dying in 1961 at the age of seventy-eight.

Of the many concepts dear to B.J., none was more so than that of innate intelligence. It was one of B.J.'s strongest premises that we ignore the most important part of ourselves, that of our own innate intelligence which controls and heals the body. By not acknowledging and working in harmony with innate intelligence, Palmer said, humanity cuts off its own right arm. He taught understanding and respect for the innate intelligence present within every human being. To him, this belief distinguished chiropractic from other healing arts and thus became the basis of chiropractic philosophy. Let's examine innate intelligence, a real truth about health.

What is it that brings life to life? One can easily tell when something is dead, whether it's a withered flower or a human body. Something is obviously missing. There is no indication of activity, no expression of life. What is responsible for this? Simply put, a life-force.

Hippocrates said that within every human being is a special in-born force. This force, power, or intelligence is contained innately within every person and automatically controls and regulates all bodily functions. Innate intelligence acts independently of our educated, conscious minds.

Palmer believed we possess two minds at birth. One is developed, already 100% functional, while the other is not. Innate intelligence is totally developed not only at birth, but even before, presiding over the conception and fetal development of every human being. The other mind, called the educated mind, starts out in life empty but begins to record and consciously act upon life's experiences.

Most of us acknowledge a wisdom that runs the universe. B.J. Palmer taught that each of us contains a part of that wisdom. Unique and different for each person, innate intelligence is what makes you, YOU. In daily life our tendency is to overemphasize the educated mind. We undervalue the innate intelligence that runs our bodies from conception. We seem to take innate for granted. Yet innate is priceless. Could you put a price tag on the power within you that keeps you alive?

Throughout his life, B.J. Palmer wrote about innate intelligence at length. He examined it and its effects. This is what he had to say on the subject:

> Many men and women have left their imprints on history without educated knowledge of the existence of a law within them, working for them. Other men and women have also left their imprints on history, believing there was such a law, that it was possibly within them, but not being conscious of any help gained from it.
>
> Then there is a small minority who have also left their imprints on history who knowingly, consciously, and understandably let the law work through them in their daily lives. Obviously, success came to all alike.

The majority, however, are without the conscious understanding of the existence of a law within themselves. This group places education as supreme and acknowledges no other source of values. They have so much education that they have no sense of understanding of anything else. In the same sense, many so-called 'ignorant' and 'uneducated' people have made superior accomplishments because of their ability to seek the law and let it work through them. They may have been shy on 'education,' but they were brilliant with knowledge and wisdom from a greater source (B.J. Palmer *Booklet #1 2 ff.).*

DUALITY OF SENSES

Let us investigate for a moment. A baby is born. That is, it comes from the womb of a woman. One side of its mental aspect knows nothing. It's little brain is vacant, nobody lives there, nobody home. It's just a great big bit of empty space—a hollow non-entity. Gradually, the five senses, which come from nowhere according to 'educated man,' begin to see, hear, feel, taste, and smell. These impressions go inward, are interpreted by what educated man doesn't know and seems to care less about. They are accumulated, card-indexed, catalogued, filed away for future use.

This baby grows, goes to kindergarten, grade school, high school, college, all the time adding to his store of impressions, called 'gaining an education.' All this time he is puffing himself up, with what he thinks he knows. All this time he is kicking down the wisdom of the ages which made him and all this possible.

Educated man, who starts with no education at birth, and piles up his theories until death, thinks he must tell God how to run the universe. So does man, who starts with no education at birth, and piles up his theories until death, thinks he must tell Innate how to run the body. Little does he realize that, no matter what he thinks, the Universe ran successfully before he was born and will continue to run successfully after he is dead. Little does he also realize that, no matter what he thinks, Innate did successfully run bodies before he was born, and will continue to run them successfully after he is dead. An intelligence wise enough to build a baby is great enough to run that baby once it is born; is great enough to run that body in all its parts including the thinking ideas it needs to exist in material form.

SOURCE — SEMI-SOURCE — NON-SOURCE

> Innate is source.
> Education is semi-source
> The body is non-source.
> Were there no source, there would be no beginning.
> Innate being the source, is the beginning.
> Education must go to Source (Innate) to have its beginning.
> The body is merely the medium of expression of Source.
> The flow is from Source to semi-source.
> And from Source to the body.
> Were there no internal source,
> where would sickness go for health?
> Where would insanity go for sanity?
> Where would the body go for life?
> Where would organs go for function?
> It is this internal source you liberate when you give an adjustment (B.J. Palmer *Booklet #1* 2 ff.). (Palmer is referring to a chiropractic adjustment which is described later.)

The following illustration is an excellent analogy of not only the philosophy behind chiropractic but also why prevention is the truest method of health care (Figure 6.1).

The sun represents universal intelligence, or God. Innate intelligence is expressed in the form of a sunbeam and our educated mind as a mirror. Regard the sun and its sunbeam as source, the mirror as non-source. The reflection is what the non-source (the mirror) reflected of the source (the sun and its sunbeam).

Is the sunbeam a part of the sun? Is the sunbeam apart from the sun? Neither. There would be no sunbeam if there were no sun and there would be no sun if it didn't have sunbeams. Therefore, there would be no innate if there were not a universal intelligence; neither would there be a universal intelligence without innates.

The educated mind is but a human mirror, its actions being but the reflections the universal intelligence gives to the brain via innate.

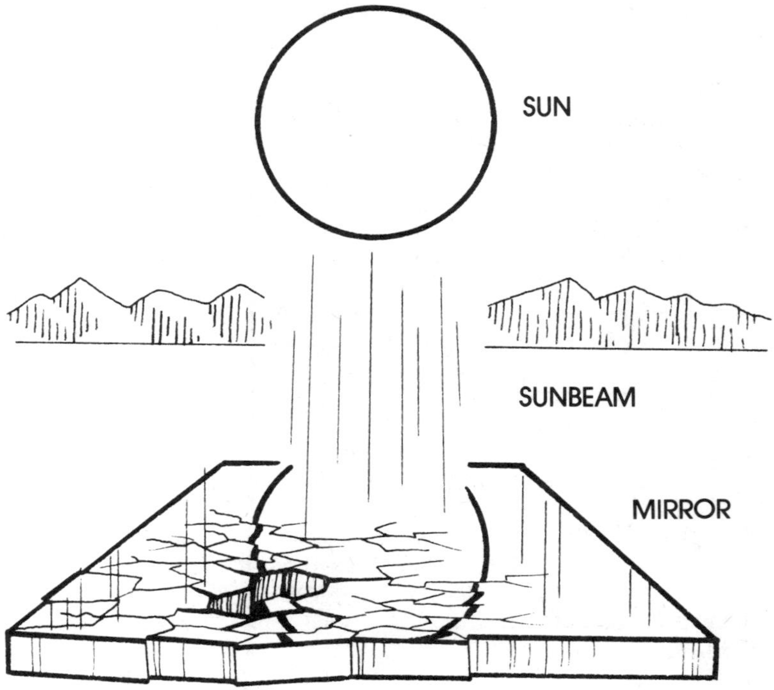

DIAGRAM OF SUN, SUNBEAM, AND REFLECTION

Figure 6-1 Adapted from Palmer, 1916

Now what if a piece of the educated mind, the mirror, is cracked as in the illustration? Can the reflection of the sunbeam (innate) off the cracked mirror be perfect? Wouldn't it make more sense to mend the mirror than to try to fix the imperfect reflection? As long as the mirror is cracked, the quality of the reflection will be reduced. As long as we treat the reflection (treating symptoms) and not the cracked mirror (treating causes), the cause is not corrected and the end result will be the same. We would understand ourselves much better and effect a greater level of health if we would pay more attention to our own innate intelligence.

On this subject, B.J. Palmer wrote in his booklet on chiropractic philosophy:

THE TRUTH

> We chiropractors work with the subtle substance of the soul. We release the prisoned impulse, the tiny rivulet of force, that emanates from the mind and flows over the nerves to the cells, and stirs them into life. We deal with the magic power that transforms common food into living, loving, thinking clay; that robes the earth with beauty, and hues and scents the flowers with the glory of the air.
>
> In the dim, dark, distant long ago, when the sun first bowed to the morning star, this power spoke and there was life; it quickened the slime of the sea and the dust of the earth and drove the cell to union with its fellows in countless living forms. Through aeons of time it finned the fish and winged the bird and fanged the beast. Endlessly it worked, evolving its form until it produced the crowning glory of them all. With tireless energy it blows the bubble of each individual life and then silently, relentlessly dissolves the form, and absorbs the spirit into itself again.
>
> And yet you ask, 'Can chiropractic cure appendicitis or the flu?' Have you more faith in a knife or a spoonful of medicine than in the power that animates the living world (15)?

The chiropractic profession as developed by the Palmers has evolved on its own and is widely practiced today. A basic understanding of a few principles utilized by chiropractors will help you understand why they do what they do. It will assist your evaluation of their abilities, enabling you to judge for yourself if they can be of help to you.

7

CHIROPRACTIC TODAY

"The doctor of the future will give no medicine but will interest his patients in care of the human frame, in diet, and in the cause and prevention of disease."

Thomas Edison

There is great social status is being a medical doctor. People don't generally think of chiropractors in the same context. Chiropractors, rather, are looked upon as separate from the medical profession. To chiropractors, that distinction is very distasteful. Many chiropractors have added other forms of therapies to their repertoire of services. They feel they have more to offer and consequently are on a par with medical doctors. They also can increase their income by providing a wider range of services.

Another reason some chiropractors render a variety of services is the lack of a specifically defined scope of chiropractic practice throughout the United States. What chiropractors should and should not practice is the most conflicting issue within the profession itself. Several different philosophies of practice have evolved through the years and often conflict with each other. This diversity has bred much apathy and lack of professional unity. Consequently, most chiropractors belong to no professional organizations.

As a result, every state in the country has a different set of guidelines governing both education and the scope of the chiropractic profession. Therefore, chiropractors seem to practice everything under the sun.

The wide range of services practiced by many chiropractors raises questions about their qualifications to practice other forms of health care, something which invokes the ethical question of trespassing into another profession's territory. A lot of friction between the medical and chiropractic professions has been created as a result. Chiropractic has failed to present its scope of practice to the medical profession, the rest of the health care community, and last but not least to us, the consumer.

Many chiropractors use only their hands in administering spinal adjustments and provide no other services to the patient. In chiropractic jargon, they are called "straights." But since the 1920's another major group, called "mixers," has emerged. They comprise the American Chiropractic Association. These chiropractors desire to practice chiropractic along with other modalities such as physical therapy and nutrition, in effect, expanding their scope of practice. Their success through the years is due to their efforts of expanding the scope of education required of chiropractors.

The disagreements between straights and mixers have caused a blight on the development of chiropractic, both as a profession and as a primary health care provider by depriving the profession of a unified identity. When you look up chiropractors in the telephone book, a variety of practices will be found using different phraseologies. Consequently, the consumer is often confused, which in turn breeds skepticism and mistrust.

Contained within the chiropractic profession are dozens of different techniques and types of practitioners to adjust the spinal column and adjacent skeletal structures. There are straight chiropractors, Hole In One (HIO) chiropractors, low-back chiropractors, full-spine chiropractors, Gonstead chiropractors, and many, many more. Some offer a very wide range of services which include forms of physical therapy, nutrition, hypnosis, accupressure, and accupuncture. Furthermore, each of the fifty states has its own laws about what chiropractors can legally do. The answers to the questions "What is chiropractic?" and "What can a doctor of chiropractic do?" are not simple.

To clarify these issues, *The Ethics of Chiropractic* by Bernard L. CiRullo D.C. discusses the field of ethics pertaining specifically to the chiropractic profession. CiRullo writes:

> There are five things which separate all trades, businesses, professions, vocations and specialties within each one of the occupations on Earth. First is a problem, disorder or disease which someone found. Second is a solution, remedy, treatment or method of operation which someone discovered to correct that problem. Third is the word, words, letters,

> abbreviations or numbers coined and used to name, confine, define, describe and explain who, what, when, where and why 'that' and not something else needs to be done. Fourth is the tool(s) or instrument(s) which someone invented to help the mind and hands find and then correct that problem, disease or disorder. And last but not least, is the school, college or university which was opened and maintained in order to teach others how to use all of the above (89).

Dr. CiRullo further explains that chiropractic as developed by the Palmers meets these qualifications:

1. D.D. Palmer discovered a disorder called a 'vertebral subluxation.'
2. He discovered a method of operation to correct that disorder, called a 'chiropractic adjustment.'
3. Nine months later he coined the root word 'chiroprac,' adding the suffixes -tic and -tor, to coin the words chiropractic and chiropractor.
4. The tools and instruments used by chiropractors began with adjusting tables D.D. Palmer made on which to lay his patients. B.J. Palmer further developed the use of X-ray equipment in 1910, heat and nerve-sensing instruments in 1921 and 1931.
5. The Palmer School (now college) of Chiropractic was opened by D.D. Palmer in 1897 (90).

Therefore, any major deviations from the above mentioned methodology would not be chiropractic. Regardless of the merit, it is unethical and misleading to the public for a chiropractor to label a wide range of services chiropractic. Chiropractic does one thing and one thing only: The locating and removing of subluxations of the spinal column through the skilled use of hands by the practitioner.

Besides the great discrepancy of services chiropractors perform, there are countless different techniques used to accomplish their primary objective: that of locating subluxations in the spines of their patients and removing them without harming the patient in the process.

Few of these techniques have been scientifically evaluated. There are a dozen major techniques being used, most developed by individuals who practiced what they discovered to be successful with their own patients. Since the profession has no unified identity, there is little sharing of techniques. Some chiropractors fear their methods will be proven ineffective. Unfortunately, it is the consumer who suffers as a result.

Chiropractors have carried a torch for years, claiming to be a separate and distinct form of health care within the healing art community. What they have actually done, though, is become separate and distinct from each other. Because the public is on the outside, few people have an intimate understanding about the inner workings of this profession. It's time chiropractors cease their intra-professional disagreements.

First, chiropractors must agree on their own identity. This will eliminate the confusion both within the profession and with the public as to what chiropractors stand for and what they are qualified to do. Next, all techniques must be scientifically tested, verified, and shared. Consumers and chiropractors alike must know which methods work and which do not.

As the field of medicine upgrades its procedures, each doctor and institution is updated, and old procedures are eliminated. Medical doctors of the 1980's don't practice 1920's medicine. The same is not true of chiropractic.

There is little policing of the techniques an individual practitioner performs on patients. It's time the people behind the techniques put their philosophical differences aside and found out who has verifiable methods and who does not.

This house cleaning won't be easy, but its time has come. These two major issues, the extent of services chiropractors can render and the manner in which they physically adjust the spines of their patients, must be resolved. This action is not to be taken as a threat to chiropractic. The biggest reason why the profession has relatively flourished is that it gets results. Often, its believers were former skeptics who turned to chiropractic when standard medical practices failed to help them. A look behind the scenes at a chiropractor's office can shed more light on this profession and the difficulties it faces.

Prior to 1975, one could be a Doctor of Chiropractic in as few as four academic years. Today requirements at most chiropractic colleges include two to four years of undergraduate study before entering a minimal four year chiropractic program. There are approximately fifteen chiropractic colleges in the

United States and another half dozen abroad.

The role of a Doctor of Chiropractic involves particular attention to the structural relationship and neurological aspects of the body in health and disease. Chiropractors' knowledge of basic and clinical sciences and other health related subjects qualifies them to analyze the spine, adjust the position of the vertebrae, care for the human body in health and disease, and consult with or refer to other health care providers. The following are several terms now used by chiropractors.

MISALIGNMENTS AND SUBLUXATIONS

The terms *misalignment* and *subluxation* are very important in understanding the condition of your spine. A misalignment occurs when your spine is out of its normal alignment but continues to function within its range of motion. A subluxation is a combination of the Latin prefix *sub-* (meaning "less than") and *luxation*, a term referring to a slight dislocation. The spine is subluxated when a vertebra is out of position in relationship with the one above or below it. As a result, the vertebra exerts pressure on the nerves that exit the spinal column between the vertebrae. This, in effect, pinches the nerves and disrupts the flow of communication between the brain and the part of the body those nerves connect (Figure 7-1).

There are four main conditions that occur as a result of a subluxation:

1. The spine is out of alignment; i.e., the position of the spinal column is no longer correct.
2. The spine is out of its normal range of motion; i.e., the position of the spinal column precludes the ability to function through a full range of motion.
3. The spine has a fixation between two or more vertebrae; i.e., the vertebrae cannot move independently of one another.
4. The spine is causing interference to the nerve impulses exiting between the vertebrae; i.e., the opening between each two vertebrae is occluded, which restricts the nerves exiting the spinal column at that point. This is the most serious consequence of having a subluxation (CiRullo 30 ff. and Leach 15 ff.).[12]

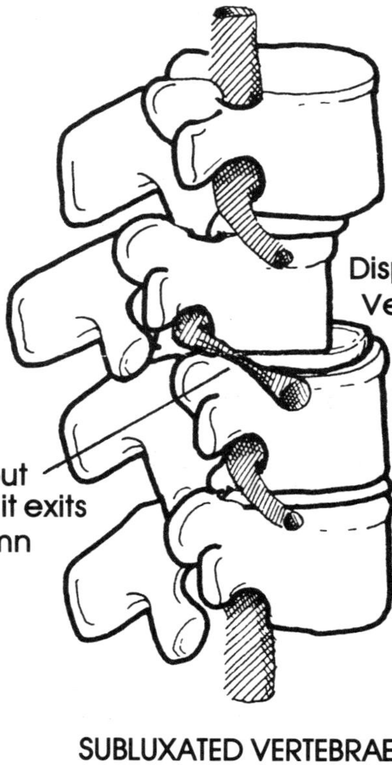

SUBLUXATED VERTEBRAE

Figure 7-1

A misalignment, though affecting the structure of the body and possibly the ability to move freely, does not affect the nerves as they exit between the vertebrae. Most subluxations, however, begin as misalignments (CiRullo 33). Putting your spine through a full range of motion several times a day eliminates the slight misalignments that normally occur and prevents them from worsening and becoming subluxations.

When vertebrae, and thus the spine as a whole, lose their proper relationship to gravity, subluxations are the inevitable result. What does it physically mean to have a subluxation?

Let's look at a simple example. When you shake someone's hand, you reach out with your arm. Your hand comes in contact with theirs. In a split second, the nerves in your hand register an impulse. That information is relayed through the nerves of your arm into your spinal cord and up to the brain. In an instant you learn a lot about the hand: how strong it is, the temperature, and so on. Then in response, your brain sends new information back through your spinal cord, out between the vertebrae of the spinal column and down the arm to your hand, all of which causes your hand to respond accordingly.

In this manner the brain constantly receives information, via the nervous system, about all functions and operations of the body, as well as external environmental stimuli. In return, it sends information back to those parts of the body, telling them what to do and how to perform. The glory of this is that you never consciously have to think about the process. The body does it innately. Subluxations interfere with this communications network. When a subluxation occurs in the spinal column, although the flow of nerve energy is blocked at that point, one often doesn't recognize it until the corresponding part of the body malfunctions and physical symptoms begin to appear.

A subluxation acts somewhat like pinching the fuel line of an automobile. The gasoline will not efficiently pass through the fuel line to the engine, causing the engine to malfunction. If the fuel line is pinched shut, the engine will soon run out of gas and cease to function altogether. Just as gasoline must flow to keep an automobile running, nerve energy must flow freely through the spine to power every part of the human body.

It's easy to understand that a subluxation in the spine can

cause problems located elsewhere in the body. The spine is our lifeline. Without proper care the spine can also be a source for many health problems. Hippocrates, the Father of Medicine, said, "Look well to the spine for the cause of disease." Understanding subluxations explains why this is so.

ADJUSTMENTS AND MANIPULATIONS

There is a vast difference between adjustment and manipulation of the spinal column and adjacent joint structures by a chiropractor. Ideally, an adjustment should be given with only as much force as necessary to move the vertebrae back into their proper alignment. NEVER should a chiropractor put more force into the body than a patient's spine can resist. Too much force can move the bones of the spinal column into an incorrect position. Creating the dynamics by which the adjustment is rendered to the patient is both an educated and intuitive process performed by the chiropractor. The innate intelligence of the patient always knows where the spinal column should be. When adjusting, the chiropractor acts only as an aid to achieving that end.

Adjustment and manipulation need to be distinguished. An adjustment is the act or action of adjusting or being adjusted. To *adjust* means to fix fast; i.e., to place at least two things in their proper positions quickly. A manipulation is the act of manipulating or being manipulated. To *manipulate* is to mold, as by a slow process of forcing something or someone to be and do that which it is not (CiRullo 31 ff.).

Physical manipulation occurs over a longer period of time, as opposed to an almost instantaneous movement of an adjustment. Regarding the spine, manipulation can result in more force being applied than the spine requires. This is called for very rarely, and then only in cases of extreme injury or serious dislocation.

Manipulation is called for in cases of dislocation injuries that occur in other areas than the spine. Manipulation largely depends on the use of the educated mind of the administering chiropractor or doctor. Adjustments, on the other hand, utilize the chiropractor's innate intelligence as well as his or her educated mind.

Adjustment of the spinal column is one of the most effective or adverse experiences that can occur to the human body. The bottom line is that you don't want your spine treated improperly.

When a chiropractor decides to move spinal vertebrae regardless of what the patient's body and innate intelligence would have preferred, that is manipulation. It can NEVER be tolerated, not even once. Adjusting the spine is akin to performing brain surgery. It is a serious and delicate process demanding the utmost competence on the part of the chiropractor.

DISEASE AND DIS-EASE

Disease means an alteration that impairs functioning of a living body. Dis-ease, on the other hand, is defined as follows: *dis* meaning "lack of," and *ease,* "comfort of mind and body." So dis-ease means lack of ease or comfort of the mind and body.

Dis-ease is an important step before disease and deals with the impairing alteration in a living body. Dis-ease means the body is not easily functioning and is how the majority of health problems begin. So by the time you detect a change in your body's condition, damage may have already taken place.

The answer is to practice health maintenance through disease prevention, which technically refers to both dis-ease and disease. This process differs from crises care, which means to do nothing or very little to maintain your health (being unaccountable), then seeking quick remedies when something goes wrong.

Chiropractors perform three main services: physical examinations (mainly muscular and skeletal in nature), X-rays (mainly of the spinal column), and adjustments of the spine. The office usually consists of a waiting or reception room, front office, insurance processing office, X-ray room, therapy rooms, and adjustment rooms. Some chiropractors also have resting rooms in which patients can lie down and relax after being adjusted. Relaxing after an adjustment helps to maintain the new position of the spinal column and allows the body time to adapt to the physiological changes that take place after an adjustment.

VISITING A CHIROPRACTOR

On the first visit to a chiropractor's office as a patient, one is usually given a health history form to complete. This form covers who you are, who is paying for your care, your health history, as well as your current symptoms and immediate concerns. Most patients spend too little time filling out these forms and as a result do not supply enough information.

The staff is trained to make sure you have all necessary financial information correctly written on the form, but the personal information about you is YOUR responsibility. It's imperative you supply all of the information completely and accurately. The chiropractor, like any doctor, benefits greatly from understanding your current condition and history in depth.

After the health history form is completed, the Chiropractic Assistant may give you literature to read. Sometimes, a slide or video presentation is shown. This acquaints new patients with the chiropractic experience. During the examination the chiropractor checks for and locates objective conditions, some of which may validate your subjective, physical symptoms.

Exams vary greatly from one chiropractor to another. Some spend several minutes, using many tests to detect overall structural and specific spinal problems. These orthopedic and neurological tests help to isolate and verify a patient's complaint. A lack of proper spinal motion is often an indicator, along with particular areas where the patient may be experiencing pain.

The examination is followed by X-rays, required by most chiropractors. How many are taken and how often varies greatly from one chiropractor to the next. Usually, one or more X-rays showing the spine from the front and from the side suffice. They can be either full spine (14'' x 36'') or smaller, more specific shots of various areas of the spine.

X-rays possess great clinical value. They allow the visual examinations of pathology and general spinal condition not afforded through touching and visual inspection with the unaided eye. Their drawback is radiation. Modern equipment, however, minimizes risk. An up-to-date, quality X-ray unit exposes the patient to an amount of radiation well within the safety standards set by the federal government.

After X-rays are taken and processed, the chiropractor analyzes them. They are generally discussed with the patient on the second visit. Sometimes the patient is adjusted on the first visit, though most chiropractors prefer to wait and see what the X-rays reveal.

On the second visit the chiropractor reports the findings to the patient. Recommendations are made for the number of office visits necessary. Any other required therapy is also discussed.

Recalling normal spinal configuration, as discussed in chapter four, can aid you in understanding your own X-rays, and therefore the condition of your own spine. This enables you to communicate intelligently with your chiropractor about your condition. It is to your advantage to find out exactly what your spinal configuration is, where your weak areas are, any pathologies you may have, and the general condition of the alignment and curvature.

Findings from the X-rays are transferred to a patient card. Each time a patient visits the office, the chiropractor refers to this card to remind himself of the patient's particular spinal configurations. It also carries information regarding adjusting methodology, the patient's progress, and any other noteworthy concerns.

Most patients are then adjusted for the first time. This procedure includes use of the fingers to feel the spinal column, also known as palpation. Often, the side and bottom parts of the chiropractor's hands are used in contact with the vertebrae. The patient is positioned on an adjusting table in a manner to control the amount of force used and the direction into the spinal column the force is going. By the process of adjusting, force extends from the chiropractor's hands into the patient's spinal column to shift the vertebrae into their proper alignment. It is imperative that the patient be relaxed and not resisting the chiropractor's movements while an adjustment is taking place.

At this point, the patient can further benefit from having a basic knowledge of the spine and avoid being at the mercy of the chiropractor's directives.

Each patient must be evaluated individually. Care shouldn't be dependent on a patient meeting a criterion that automatically results in the greatest profit for the chiropractor. The label "revolving door practice" applies when anything and everything is told to the patient to sell him or her on the idea of frequent visits. Money is the major motivation behind such practice.

The patient must realize that the chiropractor is running a business. The number of visits and types of services rendered by the chiropractor determines their income. This type of chiropractor measures profit by case average. Because of administrative costs involved with each patient, it is more profitable for the chiropractor to see fewer patients more often than more patients less often. Therefore, patients who can evaluate the number of visits prescribed in accordance to their condition can determine to whose benefit the visits will best serve.

A patient should be taught self-care and made aware of how to assist one's own healing process. Instructions are usually in the form of specific spinal exercises. Some basics are provided in the next chapter concerning proper spinal maintenance. Spinal maintenance exercises strengthen the muscles along the spine, helping to realign the spine and keep it in place.

The goal is to make patients responsible for their own care and restore them to health as soon as possible. Chiropractors utilizing these methods require fewer visits from their patients. For consumers, this is a prudent health and economic practice.

The value of any adjustment is limited when patients do not maintain their spine and remain as subluxation-free as possible. Without the patient's cooperation through exercises and proper posture, the chiropractor's adjustments are only temporary. The chiropractor must then compensate for the patient's lack of self-care and maintenance by requiring more office visits.

The techniques used by chiropractors vary greatly. Though their purpose is the same, that of removing subluxations, the mechanics often differ from one to the next. Some techniques are better at alleviating certain spinal subluxations than others. This fact further necessitates the need to scientifically evaluate chiropractic techniques. Then, depending on the patient's problem and the circumstances of the case, the right methods for correction could be utilized, eliminating a lot of guesswork.

As a supplement to adjusting, many chiropractors now use physical therapy. In certain situations, physical therapy provides great benefit to patients when administered in conjunction with spinal adjustments.

Though it is not a part of chiropractic as originally developed by the Palmers, many chiropractic colleges now teach physical therapy, an example of the expansion of chiropractic curriculum being taught.

Some states require the teaching of physical therapy because students are tested on the subject as part of the state licensing examination. Although physical therapy provides the chiropractor other methods of health care that can readily assist the patient's recovery, many learn only enough to pass the examination and are not adequately qualified to perform it on a regular basis. Consequently, physical therapy is treated as window dressing and a way to make more money.

Chiropractors practicing physical therapy should have the same qualifications as a physical therapist, medical doctor, or any other health care provider licensed to practice physical therapy. Furthermore, it should be explained to the patient that the physical therapy being performed is in fact physical therapy, not chiropractic.

Based on the technique practiced, the chiropractor decides how to adjust the spinal vertebrae. Your physical symptoms are not the only factors taken into account. Where the subluxations are located in the spine and the techniques used to remove them are what count most. There may be pain in one area but subluxations in another. Though therapy can be administered to the affected area of pain, removing the subluxations are still a chiropractor's primary concern. By the very nature of their discipline, chiropractors want to give you cause-oriented versus symptom-oriented health care.

Do not think that the more bones the chiropractor adjusts in your spine the better off you are. On the contrary, the least amount of adjustment administered by the chiropractor is best. Remember, the chiropractor is only assisting the body in healing itself. It is vital that the chiropractor knows when to adjust and when not to. Also, do not be concerned with popping or cracking sounds you may hear during an adjustment. They are not indicative of the quality of the adjustment but are the result of the suction formed when vertebrae change their position.

Some chiropractors today use machines to aid in providing specific adjustments to the spine, particularly the atlas vertebra. Although D.D. Palmer intended chiropractic to be done with the skilled use of the hands only, it is doubtful he could envision the day when a machine could become so sophisticated that it could duplicate and in some instances improve upon the ability of the chiropractor to give an adjustment.

MAXIMIZING YOUR RESULTS

Before being treated by a chiropractor, loosen your spine up thoroughly before every adjustment (as explained in chapter eight). Since patients are usually directed to an adjusting room to wait for the chiropractor, they can prepare their spine for adjustment at that time. A simple twisting exercise, shown in the next chapter, will loosen the spine and muscles of the back. Some chiropractors have a technician perform specific spinal exercises with each patient before an adjustment. This kind of preparation produces results much faster.

Sometimes patients complain that soon after leaving the office they felt their back go out of place again. This occurs when the muscles of the back are stiff and tight from not having been loosened up properly before the adjustment. Tight muscles will move the spine back out of adjustment as soon as some triggering mechanism occurs. This can be as simple as getting into your car. Be careful after receiving an adjustment not to jar your body, thus throwing your spine out of alignment again. In acute cases, patients must be particularly careful after an adjustment to do only a limited amount of movement and exercise.

If you have chronic back problems, they won't improve overnight. You might alleviate the pain a little, but the problem will remain, ready to strike again. Damage takes time to repair. Time is an essential element of healing. The more healing you need, the more time it will take.

Ultimately, chiropractors function best by helping patients prevent spinal problems from occurring in the first place.

Unfortunately, the idea of going to a doctor when you are healthy is contrary to what many of us have been taught. Prevention means maintaining the spine and having it checked periodically. This practice will catch many problems while they are minor and easily corrected.

The bottom line is, how much responsibility are you willing to take? Care of the spine is easy, and it makes sense. The brain, spinal cord, and spinal column are vital to your health. Taking care of them means taking care of you.

Taking care of your spine on a daily basis will prevent many problems from occurring in the first place. Spinal maintenance is simple and can be done in only a few minutes a day.

8

SPINAL MAINTENANCE MADE EASY

INDIVIDUALS, THROUGH INSIGHT,
DEVELOP A RELATIONSHIP WITH THEIR BODY,
FOR THE PURPOSE OF ADVANCEMENT

Since the spine is so important to our health, it's obvious we need to maintain it to remain healthy. Spinal maintenance is an easy program of self-care of the spine, utilizing inherent, innate functions of our bodies. The focus of a spinal maintenance program amounts to putting your spine through a full range of motion on a daily basis.

Notice how children are like gymnasts, very limber and agile. They can easily bend over and touch their toes. Movement for children is free and unrestricted. As many of us get older, however, we become more rigid, losing the natural elasticity of our youth. The body becomes bent over. Our range of motion diminishes. Movement in general becomes more restricted. Why does this happen?

Mechanically speaking, a major reason is that the spine has lost its proper alignment and curvature. It is therefore less capable of free and unrestricted movement. The independent movement of each vertebra of the spine is no longer possible.

Free and unrestricted movement of the spine, and therefore the body, depends on the movement of the spinal vertebrae. As long as individual vertebra are capable of independent movement, your body is able to move. Putting your spine through a full range of motion everyday will help maintain your ability to move freely and efficiently (Keim 18). Good spinal maintenance begins with determining the flexibility of your spinal column. The following indicators can be used to determine how much flexibility of motion you have.

CHECKING FOR FLEXIBILITY: THE NECK

The neck is capable of three directions of motion. The first is side-to-side motion. Normal motion means being able to turn your head to one side, positioning your chin over your shoulder, then to the other side. If you can't do that comfortably, you have lost some of the motion in your upper spine. Being able to move your head further to one side than the other also indicates a spinal problem. Your vertebrae have taken on the wrong configuration. They no longer allow the neck to move freely in one or both directions. If you start by looking straight ahead and consider that to be zero degrees, you should be able to move your head ninety degrees in both directions (Cyriax 62). (Figure 8-1).

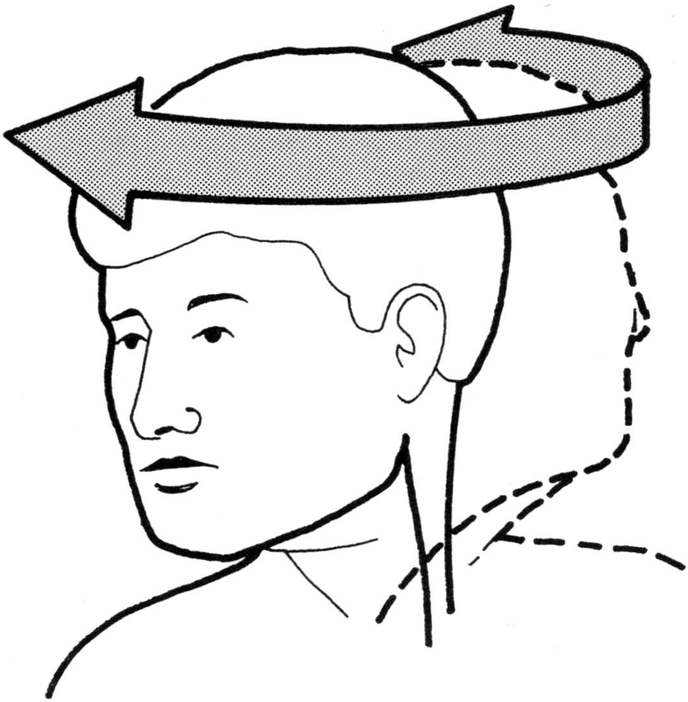

SIDE TO SIDE NECK MOTION

Figure 8-1

If you move about seventy degrees or less, you have less than normal capability. If you move between seventy-five and eighty degrees or better, some stretching may help to increase flexibility to the full ninety degrees. I caution you not to force this or any other exercise if you have a limitation or experience any pain.

The second neck motion is simply up and down, as in nodding. When you lower your chin, you should be almost able to touch it to your chest. When you raise your chin, it should point up towards the ceiling. This up and down movement should be easy and unrestricted. You should be able to raise your chin as easily as you lower it (Figure 8-2).

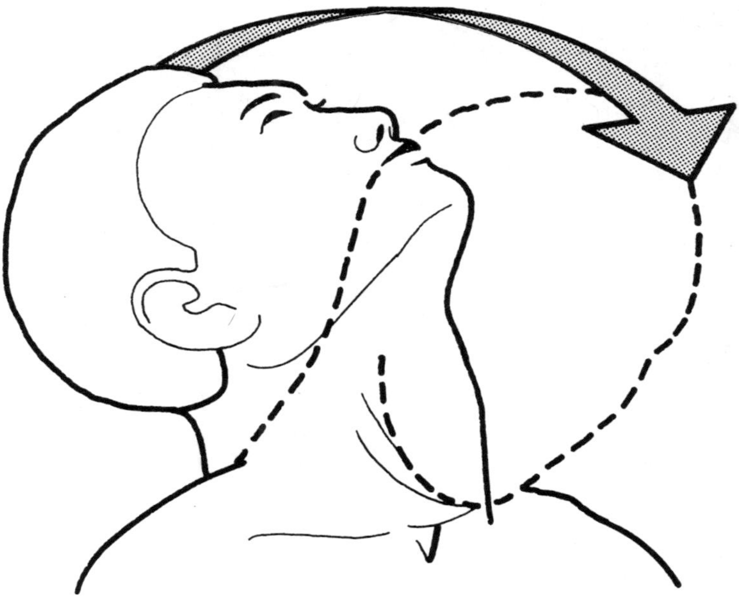

UP AND DOWN NECK MOTION

Figure 8-2

The third motion is ear-to-shoulder, that is, bringing your ear towards your shoulder while keeping your nose exactly straight ahead. Because we use the up-and-down and side-to-side movements more in everyday life, this bending motion of the neck is often neglected. You should be able to come within a few inches of your shoulder with your ear (Bourdillon 52). This is the most commonly restricted area of movement regarding the neck (Figure 8-3).

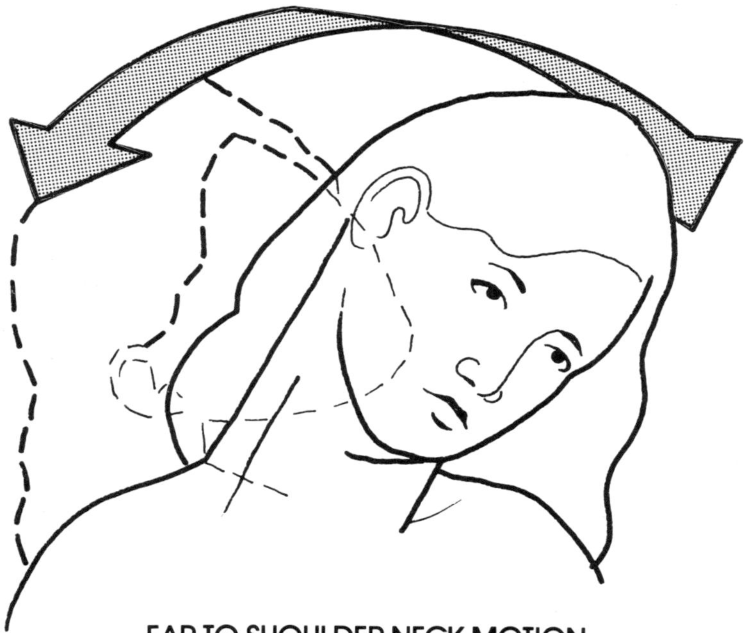

EAR TO SHOULDER NECK MOTION

Figure 8-3

CHECKING FOR FLEXIBILITY: THE LOWER BACK

The lower back has the same three motions as the neck, and by trying them one at a time, you can discover for yourself how much motion you have. The first motion is similar to touching your ear to your shoulder. Normal and unrestricted motion of the lower back means being able to slide your hands down the side of your legs to just below the knee, doing one side at a time (Steinman 36), (Figure 8-4).

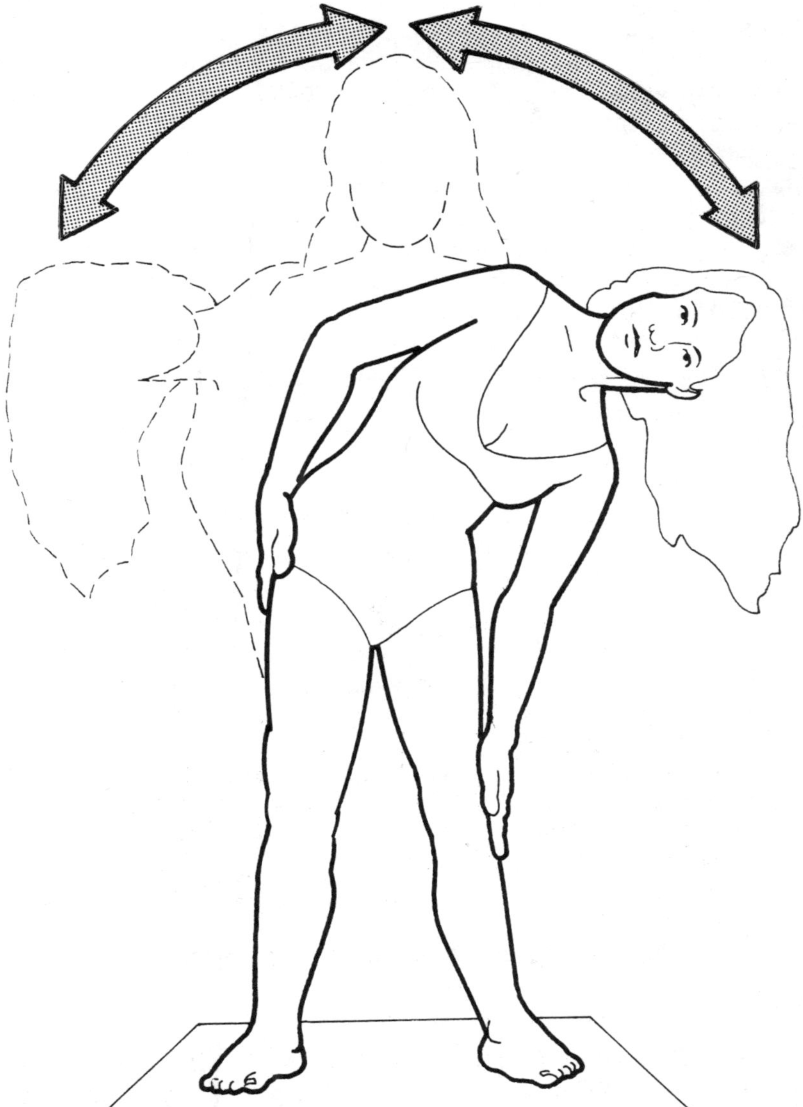

SIDE TO SIDE LOWER BACK MOTION

Figure 8-4

If doing so isn't comfortable or you can't go that far, you have lost some of the motion in your lower spine. Being able to move to one side further than the other can also indicate a spinal problem. The lumbar spine vertebrae, sacrum, or another support structure may be in the wrong configuration.

The second motion to test the flexibility of the lower back is the up and down movement of the pelvis. This action allows you to bend over and then straighten up afterwards. To begin the test, get down on your hands and knees. Then raise and lower only the lumbar spine, up and down, as if to touch your lumbar spine to the floor and when coming up, your lumbar spine to the ceiling. If you have normal flexibility, this up and down movement should be easy and unrestricted (Figure 8-5).

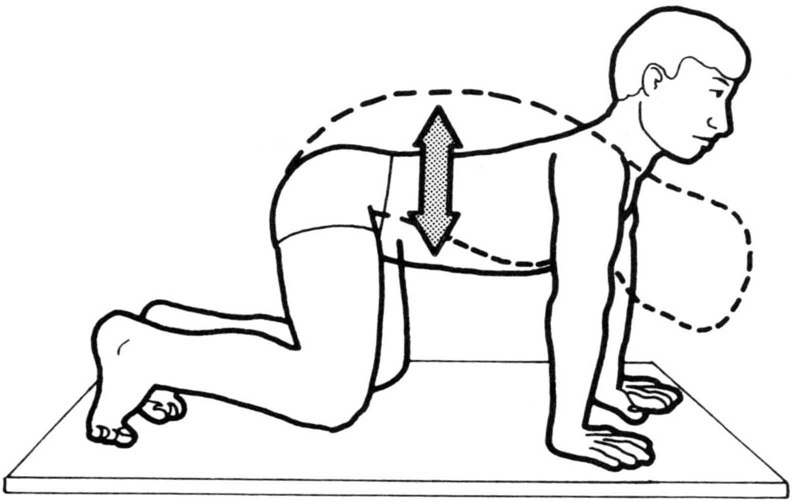

UP AND DOWN LOWER BACK MOTION

Figure 8-5

The third motion of the lower back to check is the side-to-side twisting action. While sitting, twist your upper body as far as is comfortable to one side, then the other. This motion is often used in daily life. Movement should be easy and unrestricted, and the ability to twist should be approximately the same distance to either side (Figure 8-6).

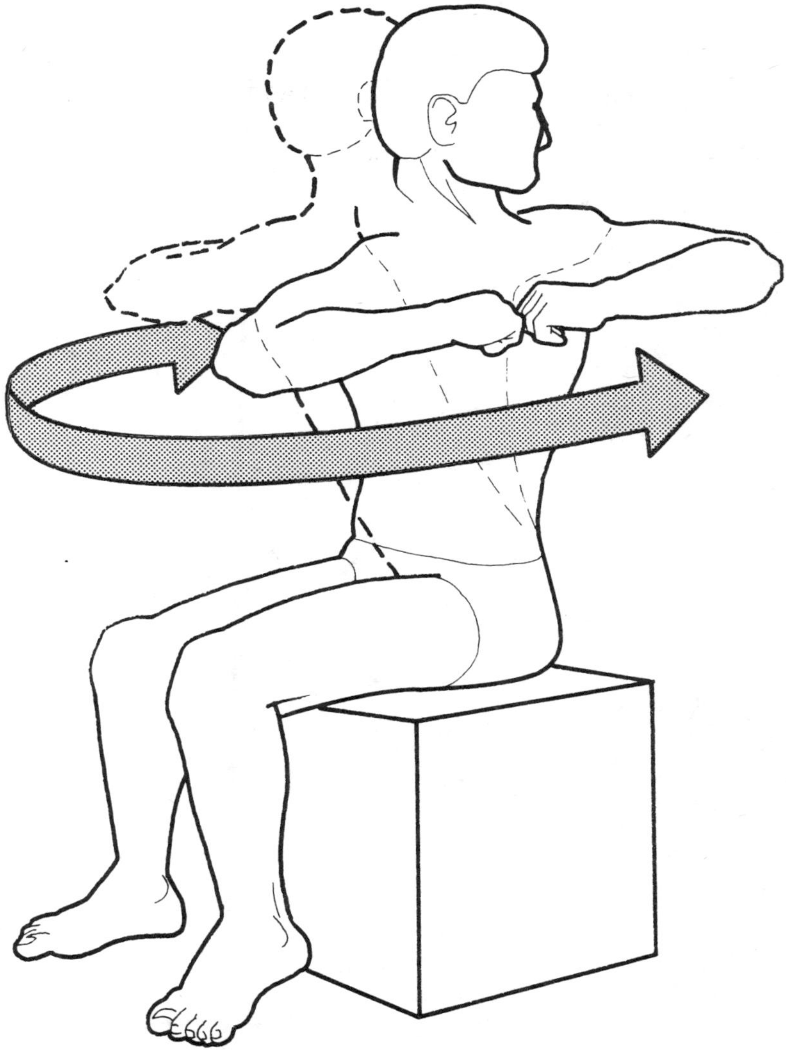

TWISTING MOTION OF THE LOWER BACK

Figure 8-6

CHECKING FOR FLEXIBILITY: THE THORACIC REGION

The other main part of the spine is the middle section known as the thoracic region. In the thoracic region, your ribs are attached to the vertebrae (Figure 8-7).

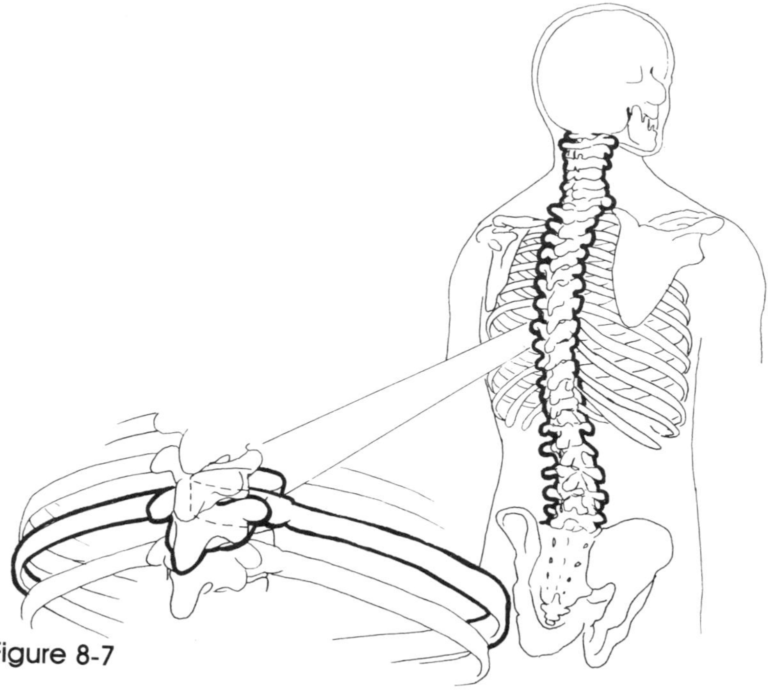

Figure 8-7

REAR VIEW OF THE THORACIC SPINE

This part of the spine is capable of much less movement and acts more as a stabilizing foundation by providing a platform for the cervical spine above and the lumbar spine below. Its main movement is a twisting, side-to-side motion. As in figure 8-6, when you twist your spine, your shoulders should turn approximately ninety degrees to either side, which is normal motion for this area of the spine (Steinman 36 ff.).

Since we have covered the basics of spinal motion, let's explore how the alignment of the spine is involved in daily life.

THE SPINE AND DAILY MOVEMENT

When the spine is out of alignment, so is the rest of the physical structure of the body. Misalignment of the spine puts other joints at a disadvantage. When they are not in proper alignment, problems can result, and until the cause of the stress is removed, the condition is unlikely to improve. Your back and your body will begin to wear out faster. Let's take the way we walk as an example.

Many people have a unique style of walking which reveals the condition and position of their spinal column. It also speaks greatly about their overall condition and personal attitude. For example, some people walk as if they carry the weight of the world on their shoulders. Their health and outlook on life is often less then optimal.

Your weight, the force of gravity, and the forces you put into your body while walking produce stress on your spine. This stress compounds any structural problems you may have. For example, since the legs are connected to the spine at the hips, misalignment of the spine can cause one hip to be higher than the other. Therefore, one leg becomes shorter than the other, and distribution of body weight becomes unbalanced. One side has more weight and force to contend with than the other. That side of the body will deteriorate faster, just as a tire wears out when the front end of a car is out of alignment (Rowe 52).[13] The loss of spinal column integrity is an identifiable cause of breakdown in a person's physical frame.

Just as there are standards by which to evaluate your spine regarding motion, strength, and construction, so too are there indicators that reflect the body's level of wellness. Take height, for example.

When was the last time you measured yourself? Often, as people become older, they become shorter. This is considered normal. Show me a person who is the same height or within a half inch of what he or she was at maturity. That person is probably someone who still stands up straight. This is not to be confused with the fact that as most of us get older, the discs in our spine shrink slightly and the cumulative effect means an overall reduction in height. I am referring to the loss of spinal column integrity resulting in a person being stooped over or otherwise no longer standing straight.

Doesn't it seem that people who stand the straightest are also in good health? They tend to be more active and have fewer aches and pains. Because they maintain good posture, they use more of their total lung capacity as opposed to a person who is bent over. They are stronger and capable of a greater range of motion. Because their joints suffer less wear and tear, people who maintain good posture throughout life will be able to get around and adequately fend for themselves at an advanced age. They will enjoy life longer and not be dependent upon others for their daily care.

Remember, gravity pulls the body down. It's a constant force all through life. If we succumb to it and can no longer stand straight, a corresponding decline in our ability to function well and experience life fully results. We gradually do less and less, until we become limited to the point of dependency. That's why physical exercise and motion are so necessary to maintain health. If your motion becomes limited and you can't move your spine, you can't exercise. If you can't exercise, your health will almost certainly begin to decline.

The spine controls our capability for motion and painless movement. Daily activities generate forces that go directly into the spine. It is important to understand that the biggest challenge we face is integrating this information into our lifestyles. The spinal column integrates all structural parts of the body, both internally and externally. Understanding what the body automatically does every day to keep us going is both incredible and inspiring. To maintain or improve your health, certain things MUST be done.

One more element important to understanding the spine is stress. Most of your stress is felt along your spine. Stress is held between your shoulders, in your head, or in your lower back. Stress, like air, is everywhere. We carry it throughout life. The effect stress has on our health depends on how we adapt to it. Unless you take action to alleviate stress, it can contribute to the deterioration of your spine over the course of your life.

This covers the main reasons why care of your spine is so important. All of the evidence points in that direction.

These problems can not only be corrected, but they can also be prevented. It just takes ACTION—simple and effective action on your part. Let's examine how easy it is to take care of your spine.

SPINAL STRETCHING AND TWISTING

Our bodies possess certain automatic, innate abilities and functions: breathing, healing, eliminating waste, and so on. We accomplish these without conscious thought. Another important built-in function is our desire to stretch. What do babies do upon awakening? They stretch. They loosen themselves up and get ready to move. Babies stretch the whole body: Hands open and close, arms and legs move back and forth. Likewise, look at an animal in nature or your own dog or cat. They also stretch upon awakening.

Although stretching is instinctive, particularly the first thing in the morning, we seem to lose the habit somewhat as we go through life. We can use that instinct in a productive manner by simply taking a moment to stretch with a purpose in mind. Many injuries could be prevented by properly stretching the body, especially the first thing in the morning and before any strenuous activity.

Preparing yourself for each day is a necessity. With all the tensions and exertions of modern life, some daily preparation of your physical body is essential. Stretching your spine prepares your body physically for the activities it will undergo during the day. Doing so is simple common sense which guards against losing your ability to have a full range of motion. And your body's motion, you'll recall, depends upon the spine.

Unfortunately, our modern lifestyle can be very damaging to the spine. What happens when the alarm goes off in the morning? We jump out of bed, hop into the shower, stuff something into our mouth on the way out the door, battle traffic all the way to work, and hope we get there with a minute or two to spare. No time has been spent on the spine and body to warm them up and properly prepare them to cope with the stresses of the day. How many people hurt themselves just getting out of bed, out of the shower, or into the car in the morning? Most injuries of this type can be avoided if the spine is properly warmed up.

Take a minute to put your spine through its full range of motion several times daily. Remember the old adage "Use it or lose it." This is another truth about health.

The most effective exercise for care of the spine is called "spinal twisting." Perform this exercise in a seated position which will keep your hips stationary and prevent them from rotating from side to side. Raise your arms to shoulder level. Put your hands directly in front of your chest.

Now SLOWLY twist to one side and then the other, moving your head comfortably back and forth also. As you do this a few times, you will feel your spine loosen. As it becomes more flexible, you will be able to move further to each side (Figure 8-8).

Doing the spinal twisting exercise involves no movement below the waist; this is strictly a torso exercise. Think of moving your head, neck, shoulders and arms together the way a washing machine does in the gentle cycle: Back and forth, back and forth. Movement should be deliberate but not jerky. If you get light-headed, you're going too fast. Twisting from one to two minutes at a time provides maximum benefits.

NEVER force your spine to go further than it is comfortably able to. When first starting this exercise, some stiffness may be felt. The stiffness is often attributable to your spine's lack of utilization of its full range of motion. If the motion of your spine in twisting is limited or painful, you may have a spinal problem. Pain is your body's way of telling you something is wrong. Listen to your pain. You may need to seek professional assistance.

Spinal twisting can also help you measure how much motion your spine is capable of, working as a unit, as opposed to each part or curve. From a seated position, pick a spot at eye level that is a few feet directly behind you. After loosening up your spine, by twisting it, you should be able to see that spot as easily from both sides as you turn back and forth. Movement to either side should be approximately the same amount. You are putting your spine through a full range of motion. There should be no pulling, straining, or forcing the body. If the spine doesn't naturally go that far, again, don't force it.

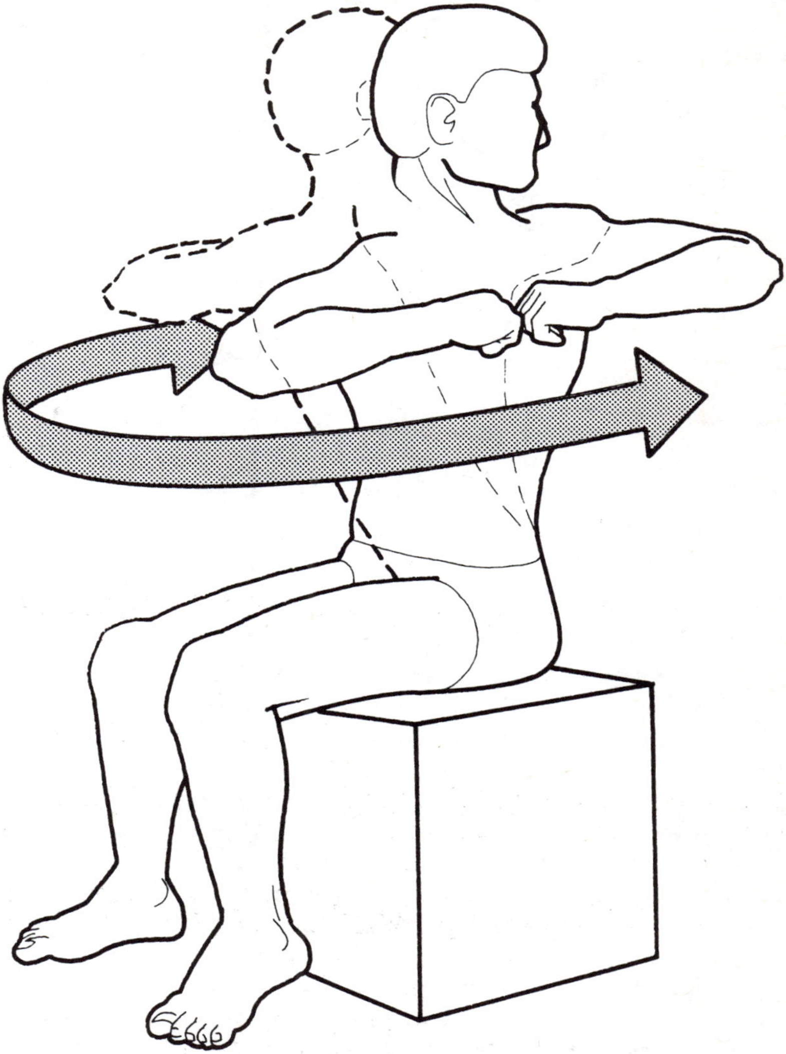

SPINAL TWISTING EXERCISE

Figure 8-8

Spinal twisting can also be done lying down. In bed or on the floor, lie on your back with your arms outstretched. Keeping your feet flat, bring them up to your buttocks. Then turn your head to one side and your legs to the other. The movement should be slow and easy. Your legs and head should reach the halfway point (pointing straight up) at the same time (Figure 8-9).

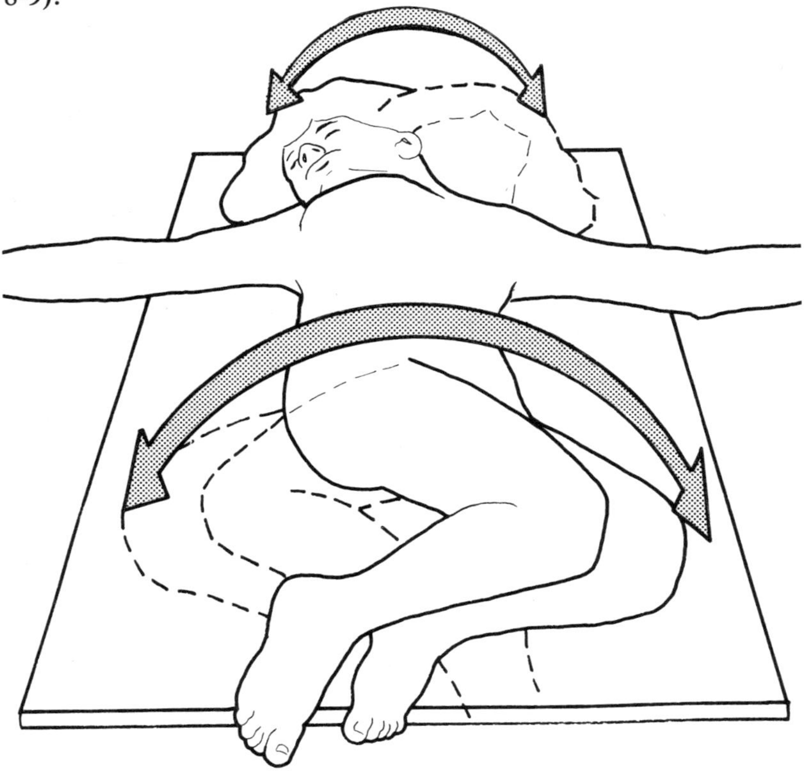

SPINAL TWISTING DONE LYING DOWN

Figure 8-9

Twisting your spine, whether in a seated or reclining position, is important. It is one of the most effective exercises you can do for yourself physically. If you aren't going to do any other exercise, at least twist your spine. This is the part of your body that must move first each time you want to change your physical position.

Other good times to twist your spine are after you have been sitting in one position for a while, such as when getting out of a car, watching TV, or following any period of inactivity. You know how stiff your back can feel after sitting or having the spine in the same position for a period of time. This is partially due to how the spine normally functions.

When you stay in any position for very long, such as bending over, your back can become stiff, making straightening up again difficult. Supporting your body weight takes a lot of energy. When you are stationary for a few minutes, the body senses this lack of activity and takes measures to conserve your energy. Energy is conserved by allowing the muscles along your spinal column to relax. The spinal column becomes rigid, assuming more of the task of supporting your body. The spinal column is then taking on the configuration your body is in.

To conserve energy, your spine automatically conforms to any position it is in for more than a few minutes. That's why cradling the telephone receiver on your shoulder puts an uncomfortable kink in your neck. It's an unnatural configuration for your spine. This happens anytime you are in an unusual posture for very long. The body should maintain correct posture when it is in a resting position. When it isn't, the muscles and/or vertebrae can be forced into the wrong position and out of normal alignment.

Many injuries occur as the result of not properly preparing the spine for movement. Save yourself from grief. Twisting the spine is easy to do and takes only a minute or two.

DEVELOPING AND MAINTAINING SPINAL CURVATURE

We can now take this information about the spine and its proper care one step further. An adjunct to the spinal twisting exercise is preparing the spine for sleep. Sleeping performs many functions. It is a time for the entire body to relax, both mentally and physically. It is also an important time for the body internally to rest as well as cleanse and repair itself.

During sleep, the body does the majority of its repair work, replacing sick or dying cells with new cells. It is vital that, while sleeping, the spine is in proper alignment. When you first go to sleep, the body instinctively attempts to remove the kinks and misalignments in your spine that build up during the day. This is done to correct and maintain proper spinal alignment, which in turn provides for the unrestricted flow of nerve impulses through the spine to every part of the body.

This natural process of correcting spinal alignment may interfere with normal sleeping patterns. You may find yourself tossing and turning, trying to get into a comfortable position for your body to rest in. The body will expend energy all night if it has to, trying to realign the spine at the expense of getting a good night's sleep and performing other vital functions as well. Therefore, you will sleep better and help your own internal healing processes by preparing the spine before you go to sleep.

Preparing your spine for sleep first involves loosening your spine thoroughly by twisting. Then lie with rolled towels under your neck and lower back to shape and mold your spine, allowing it to regain and maintain its proper curvature and alignment.

Use either a hand towel or a small bath towel. First, fold it in half lengthwise. Then bring the two sides to the middle, leaving a slight gap between them. Then roll up the towel. The gap in the middle of the towel provides a slight depression where the bony part of the back of the vertebrae, called the spinous processes, will rest. Place rubber bands at both ends of the towel to keep it together (Figure 8-10).

By lying on the towels, you are controlling the position in which your spine will relax and the shape it will assume. As a result, your sleep time is spent with your spine in its proper and most restful position (Cardoso 92 ff.), (Figure 8-11).

This practice re-establishes proper spinal alignment and curvature. It eliminates the striving for normal position that often occurs during sleep.

When using the towels, it is important to check their correct size and placement. Lie face-up on your bed or other flat and firm surface. Place the rolled up towel under your neck below the ears. The back of your head must touch the surface on which you lie. If your head does not, the towel is too large and

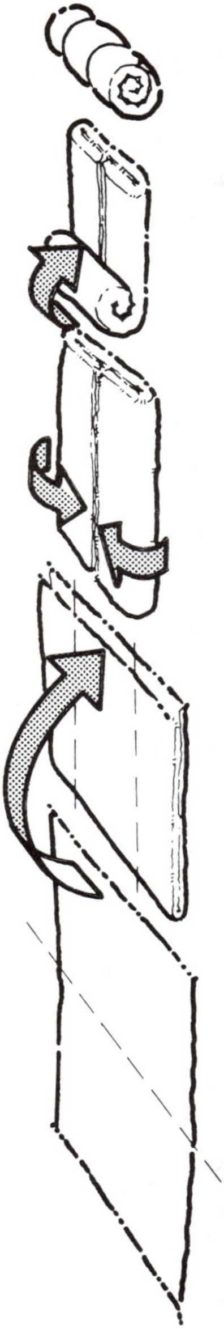

Figure 8-10

PREPARATION OF TOWEL

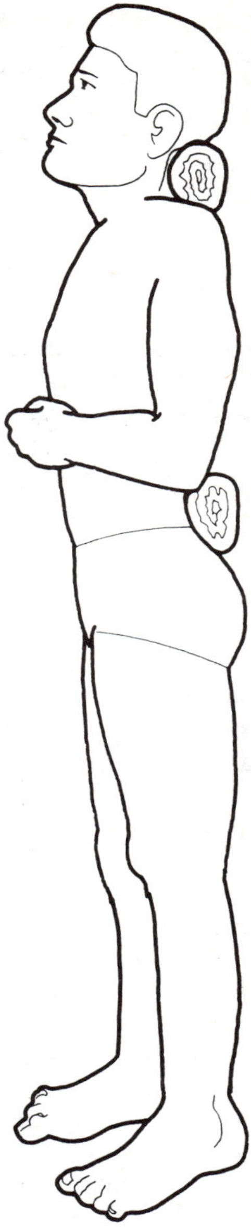

Figure 8-11

USE OF TOWELS IN SPINAL MAINTENANCE

you'll put a kink in your spine. Next, make sure the towel is not too small.

The towel is too small if you can spin it around with your hands while you are lying on it. A towel that is too small will not promote curvature. You also have to consider the firmness of the surface you are lying on. The softer the surface, the bigger the towel you will need since the towel tends to sink into a soft surface. Experiment to see what is best for you. Make sure the size and placement are correct. If they are not, the exercise won't be beneficial.

The lower back towel functions in exactly the same way as the one under the neck. It will promote and maintain the curve of the lower back. By doing the twisting exercise prior to using the towels, you make sure that the lower back is properly loosened. Again, you may have to experiment with the size of the towel.

The lower back towel should be placed so that it is right in the middle of the lower back curve. Think in terms of placing your hands on your hips. The top of either hip bone is known as the iliac crest. In this area of your back is where the towel belongs.

Your buttocks should touch the surface you are lying on, and your lower back should feel comfortable. If the towel is too small, you won't feel it under you. If it is too large, your buttocks may not be lying flat on the surface of the bed, and your lower back may feel forced up too high.

In cases in which a person has less than normal curvature, it may be necessary to increase the size of the towel as normal curvature returns. The goal is NOT to continually increase the size of the towel, but rather to reach normal curvature for your spine and maintain it.

You will have reached your normal curvature when using a larger towel becomes uncomfortable. The size of the towel should remain constant at this point.

It is important to use common sense when performing this or any other spinal exercise. Spinal maintenance, as well as any other form of self-help, requires working in harmony with your mind and body, being aware of what they are telling you.

Ideally, lie on the towels up to twenty minutes. You do not have to fall asleep on them. In fact, it is not recommended that you sleep on the towels at first since your spine may need some time to get used to them. With repetition you will find the procedure very restful.

How often can you use the towels? As often as you wish. Besides using towels before going to sleep at night, they can be used any time you take a rest. Lying on them every night would be best, but even once or twice a week is better than not at all.

There are a few things to consider when deciding how often is right for you. Definitely, the more you use the towels, the more they will benefit you. If you twist your spine before going to sleep, your body can better tolerate a night without the towels. The key is to twist the spine thoroughly at first, thereby preparing it to cool down and relax in its proper alignment.

This use of towels, like the twisting exercise, can be useful to virtually everyone. Only those with definite spinal problems will have difficulty and should not use them unless prescribed for their condition by their doctor or chiropractor. If you try using the towels and experience pain or don't feel any better, either you are not loosening your spine beforehand, you are placing the towels incorrectly, or there may be something wrong with one or more parts of your spine. In that case, discontinue the use of the towels.

These are common sense methods which can be easily integrated into one's life to get the most results. You and your body are designed to work together. Bodily harmony is another truth about health.

9

BASIC SPINAL EXERCISES AND TERMINOLOGY

"Better to hunt in fields, for health unbought,
than fee the doctor for a nauseous draught.
The wise, for cure, on exercise depend;
God never made his work for man to mend."

John Dryden

We have discussed the spinal twisting exercise, the use of towels, and preparing the spine for sleep. These procedures are the foundation of good spinal maintenance. The following exercises are designed to put each section of the spine through its full range of motion. They include exercises for the three types of movement for the neck and lower back. An exercise which helps to maintain proper alignment, flexibility, and strength of the thoracic part of the spine is also included.

EXERCISING THE NECK REGION

The spinal twisting exercise previously discussed included the side-to-side rotation of the neck (refer to figure 8-6). The second neck motion requires moving the head up and down. To do this exercise, begin by looking straight ahead. Slowly lift the head raising your chin as high as is comfortable. Then lower the chin, attempting to touch it to your chest. After several repetitions, you will notice an increasing ease of motion and be able to cover more distance. This movement, done a few times throughout the day, develops and properly maintains curvature in your neck (Figure 9-1).

The third exercise for the neck is ear-to-shoulder, that is moving your head down to one side and then the other, as if to touch your ear to your shoulder. This exercise should be done after the other two. It's important that the neck be as loose as possible before beginning. Start by looking straight ahead, keeping your nose pointed forward, Then lay your head to one side. Only go as far as is comfortable. Do the same thing on the other side. Do

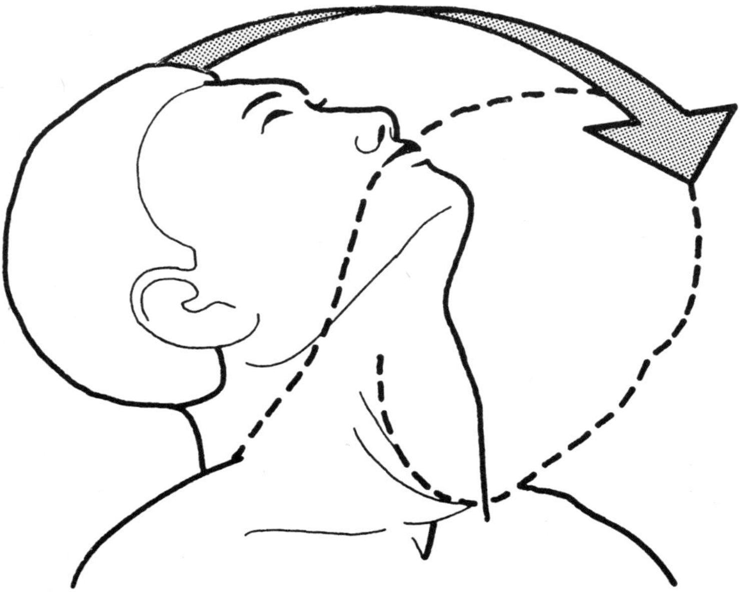

EXERCISING UP AND DOWN MOTION OF THE NECK

Figure 9-1

not raise your shoulders as you move your head. They should be completely stationary. Be aware of not turning your chin to either side as you perform this exercise (Figure 9-2).

Perhaps because it's the least used of the neck's movements, many of us have more stiffness in this dimension of movement than in the other two. It may take time to develop proper motion in this exercise. Normal motion means being able to position your ear within approximately two inches of your shoulder. After having completed this and the preceding two exercises, you have now put your neck through its three ranges of motion.

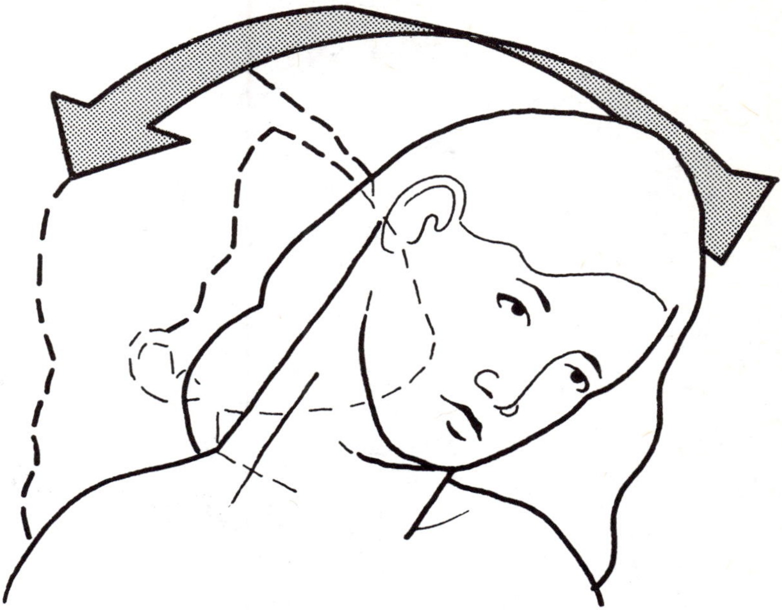

EXERCISING EAR TO SHOULDER MOTION OF THE NECK

Figure 9-2

EXERCISING THE THORACIC REGION

After the neck, the thoracic (middle) region of the spine also requires stretching and maintenance of flexibility. In the thoracic region, side-to-side motion is handled by the spinal twisting exercise. The following is a general exercise for the front to back motion of this region. Either sitting or standing, raise your arms forward above your head and press the palms together while taking a deep breath. While holding that breath, bring your hands down in front of your chest while arching the middle of your back out. Do not use a lot of force. Lean forward slightly to help the arching of the curve in the midback. Count to five and then exhale (Figure 9-3).

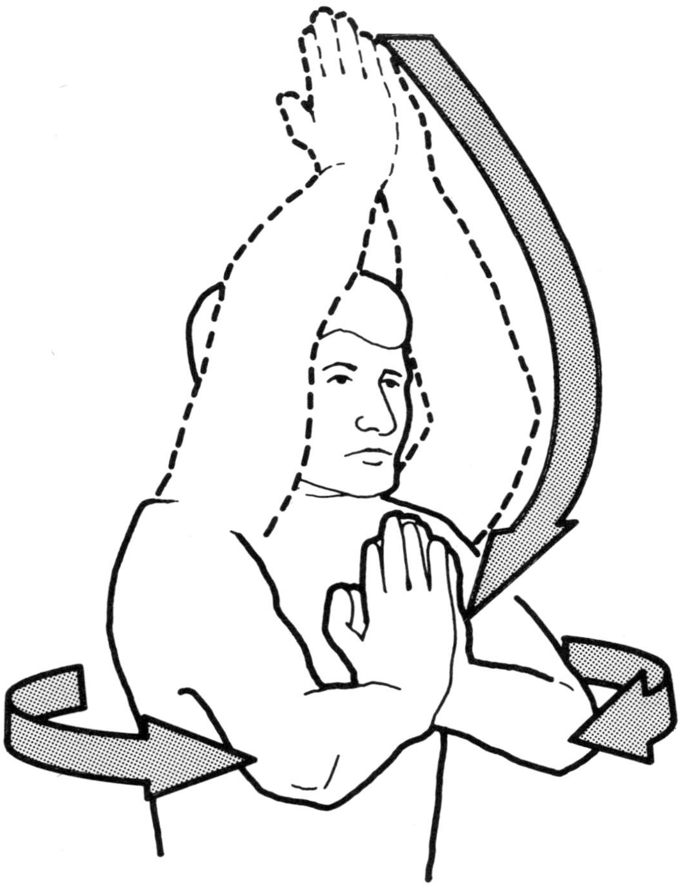

THORACIC STRETCHING EXERCISE

Figure 9-3

As a complement to this exercise, stretching the thoracic region in the opposite direction is accomplished by bringing your arms back behind the body, attempting to touch your shoulder blades together. While doing this, push your chest out. Do this while keeping your upper body relaxed. Do not flex your arm muscles. Keep them relaxed and merely rotate your shoulders backwards (Figure 9-4).

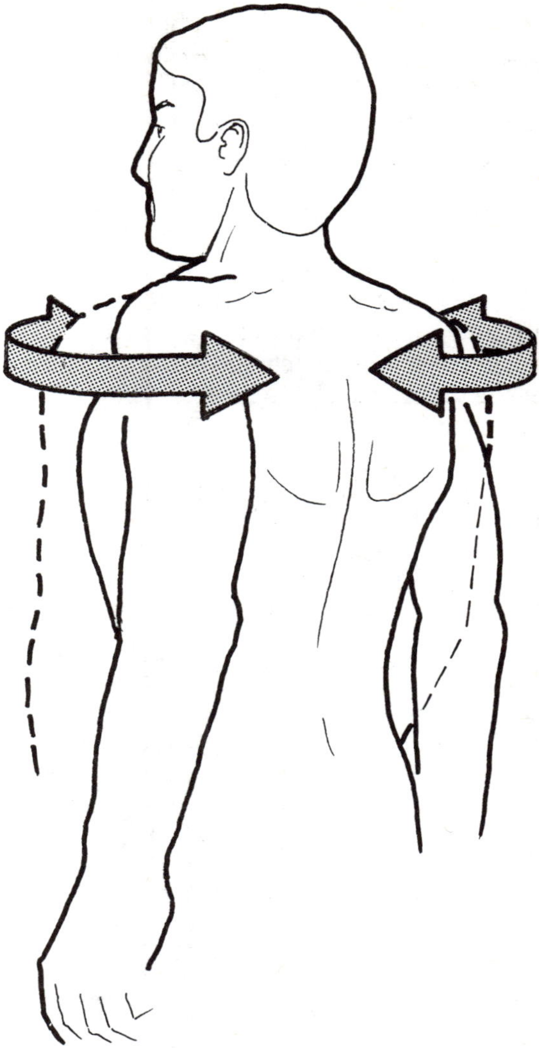

TOUCHING SHOULDER BLADES

Figure 9-4

EXERCISING THE LOWER BACK REGION

Exercising the lumbar or lower region of the spine follows the same three motions as the neck exercises. Exercising the side-to-side rotation is done by doing the spinal twisting exercise on the floor. First, lie face-up on the floor or a firm bed. Keep your feet flat on the surface and bring them up to the buttocks or as high as is comfortable. Extend your arms. Turn your head to one side and your legs to the other. The motion should be slow and smooth.

You are twisting the upper part of the spine in one direction and twisting the lower part in the other. Do it gently at first. Then, as your body relaxes, you can go further to each side. Your legs and head should reach the halfway point (pointing straight up) at the same time (Figure 9-5).

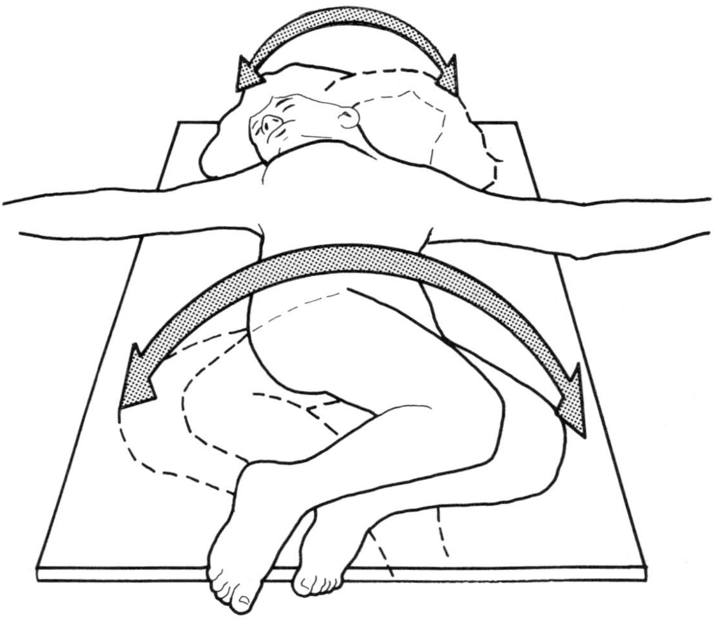

SPINAL TWISTING DONE LYING DOWN

Figure 9-5

The next exercise, called the cat stretch, is for front to back motion of the lower back, and is particularly beneficial for pregnant women. It is commonly shown to people who don't have a lot of flexibility in their lower back, a condition which may be contributing to their back problems.

Begin by getting down on your hands and knees. Keep your arms and legs perpendicular to the floor. In this exercise, only your hips and lower back move. You are, in essence, moving only your lower back up and down. The arms and upper body remain still.

This exercise is not like push-ups because the arms do not bend. You simply move your lower spine up and down, very gently at first, until it is fully relaxed. In the forward or downward motion, lower your stomach toward the floor. Then move it in the opposite direction until your back is arched like that of a cat. Inhale as you lower your body; exhale as you raise it (Figure 9-6).

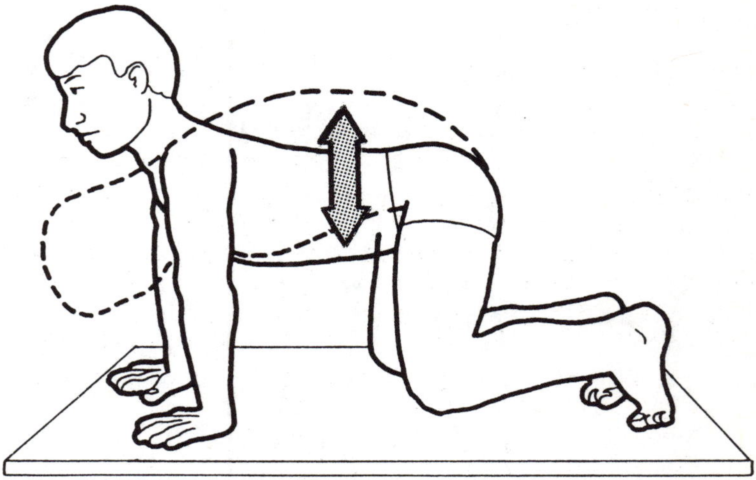

EXERCISING UP AND DOWN MOTION OF THE LOWER BACK

Figure 9-6

The third motion of the lower back is from side-to-side and is performed quite easily. Begin in a standing position. Then bend to one side, reaching your hand as far down the side of your leg as is comfortable. Repeat the exercise to the other side (Figure 9-7). Remember to start slowly and don't force yourself. Go only as far as is comfortable. A similar exercise can be done lying down.

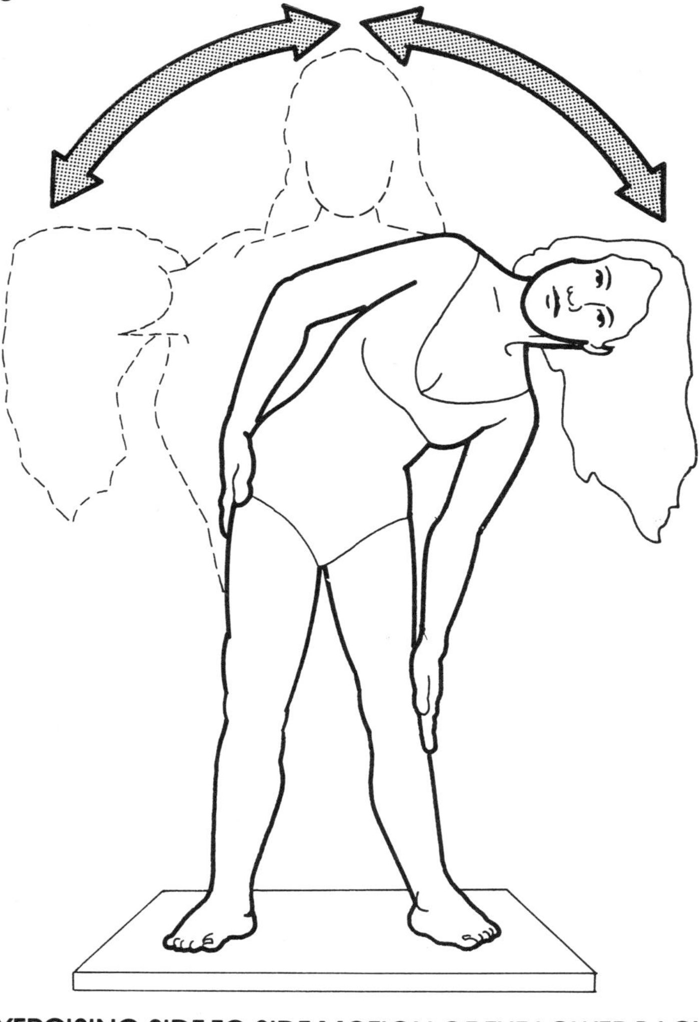

EXERCISING SIDE TO SIDE MOTION OF THE LOWER BACK

Figure 9-7

Lie down on a firm surface, face up. Cross one leg over the other at the ankles. Then, keeping your legs on the surface, drag them to one side. Keep your hips flat while performing this. Now drag them back to the other side. Uncross your legs. Put the other leg on top. Drag your legs over to the other side as far as is comfortable. Now drag them back again (Figure 9-8). These general exercises will complement the two master spinal care exercises, twisting and the use of the towels.

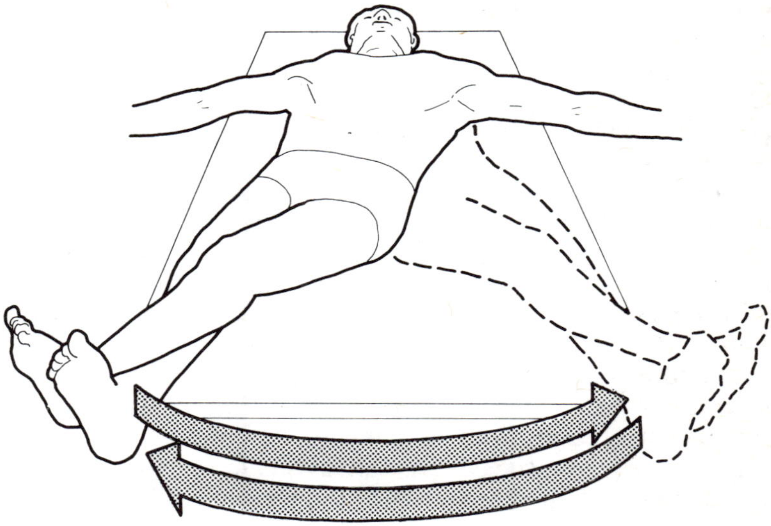

LEG DRAG EXERCISE

Figure 9-8

SUBLUXATION CONFIGURATION

The term subluxation configuration refers to the physical shape your spine takes once it's clearly out of normal position. Most spines have the tendency to go out of alignment in the same place. This is like a weak link in a chain. Each time the spine is subjected to more force or stress than it can handle, it will slip out of position in that spot, usually into the same or similar configuration each time. People will say, "My back always bothers me in the same place." The discomfort from this situation may also include getting a headache and/or pain between the shoulders or in the lower back. This condition can occur repeatedly.

When your spine has deviated from normal alignment in any one place for a long period of time, a permanent problem can develop in that area. As the weak area of your spine, that area becomes your structural Achilles' heel. Often, this is the result of subluxations which have been present for years, but which were left untreated. The best way to prevent these kinds of problems is to keep your spine in proper alignment, exercising it daily and warming it up before doing anything strenuous. If you already have a recurring problem, a qualified professional can teach you to do specific spinal exercises. Exercise counterbalances those forces that cause the spine to go out of its normal alignment.

Understand that no two people have spines with exactly the same shape. What is normal and characteristic of your spine may not be for others. There are, however, fundamentals involved with understanding a normally positioned spine.

The spine can be understood in relation to gravity (Pettibon *Theory* 38). This refers to the perpendicular stance of the human body. Gravity always pulls the body down. How straight the spinal column is (viewed front to back) in relation to gravity provides an accurate measurement of its condition and areas that are under excessive stress. Deviations in the spinal column can be measured in degrees of rotation away from the up and down center line or midline of the body (Pettibon *Theory* 74).

Under normal conditions, our tolerance level is approximately half to one and a half degrees to one side or the other. After that, the ability to move is affected, and we begin to disrupt the nervous system itself. Additionally, the curves of the spine, (the spine being viewed from the side) can be measured to evaluate their condition and the relative strength factor of the spinal column itself (Pettibon *Spinal Model* 9 ff.). There are specific relationships between the various skeletal structures of the body. The alignment of each structure is understood in relationship to the ones adjoining it. Finding the midline of your body and how closely you are aligned to it starts with your skull.

You find the center of your skull mass by bisecting it. The

center of your skull mass should be ninety degrees in relation to the atlas, the top vertebra of the spine on which the skull rests. The skull and atlas meet at the foramen magnum. This is a large opening at the base of the skull where the spinal cord exits the brain and enters the spinal column. The atlas has two concave lateral masses that fit the convex condyles of the skull (Figure 9-9).

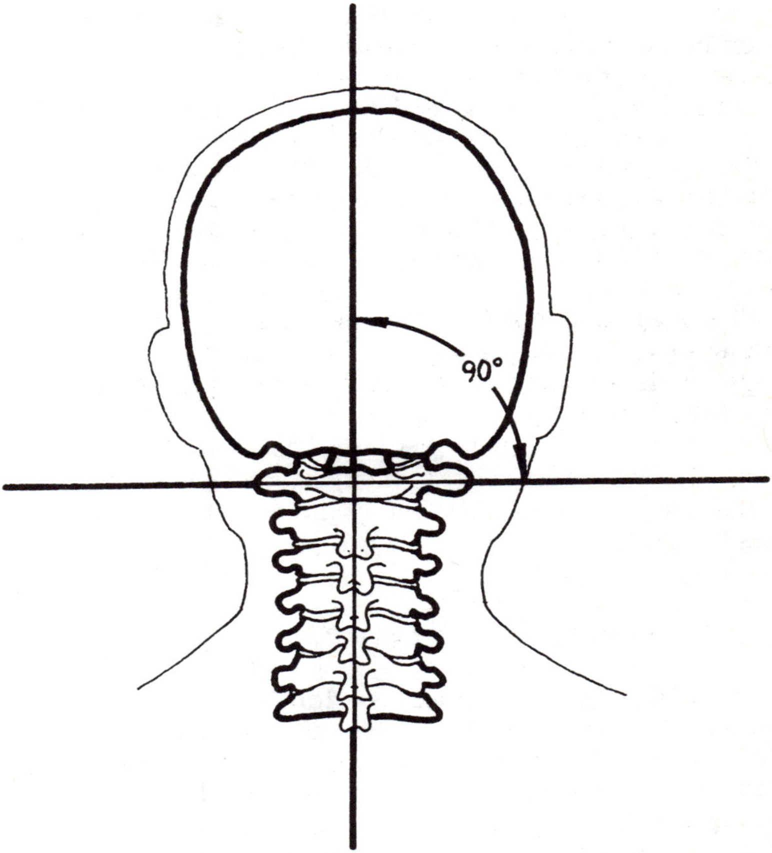

BISECTING THE SKULL

Figure 9-9

The atlas vertebra is specifically designed to transfer the skull mass (approximately ten pounds for an average adult) onto the top of the cervical spine. The atlas is the most important vertebra in your spine. It should be perpendicular to the skull.

When the atlas is not perpendicular to the skull, it can affect the flow of nerve impulses through the rest of the spinal column and thus, the rest of your body. The atlas has more freedom of movement than any other vertebra of the spine.

The second cervical vertebra, the axis, has a vertical projection called the odontoid. It centers the rotation of the movement of the atlas (refer to Figure 4-9).

In a front-to-back view of the spine, the spine should be straight up and down. There should be little, if any, deviation. When viewed from the side, the curves can be measured in degrees. Engineering principles tell us that the strongest curve, or arc, is one that has a radius of curve equal to the chord across the arc. This principle also applies to the spine (refer to Figure 4-3).

Through the use of formulas and measurement, the extent or value of one's spinal curve can be accurately measured. The spine itself is structured so that the cervical curve of the neck plus the lumbar curve of the lower back equals the thoracic curve of the middle spine (Pettibon *Theory* 40 ff.). The gain or loss of curvature anywhere in the spine, along with the resultant compensation taking place within the rest of the spine, can be easily detected.

VISUAL SPINAL EXAMINATION

There is a simple test to see how straight the atlas is in relation to the rest of the spine. Have the person being tested stand facing you. People with proper alignment of their atlas vertebra in relationship with the rest of their spine should be able to look straight ahead at you, close their eyes, slowly turn their head from side to side, then return to the same position from which they started. When they open their eyes they should be looking in the same position they were when the test began, directly at you. If it is obvious that their head is turned to one side or the other, their neck is not in proper alignment (Figure 9-10). One can also perform this exercise by themself in front of a mirror.

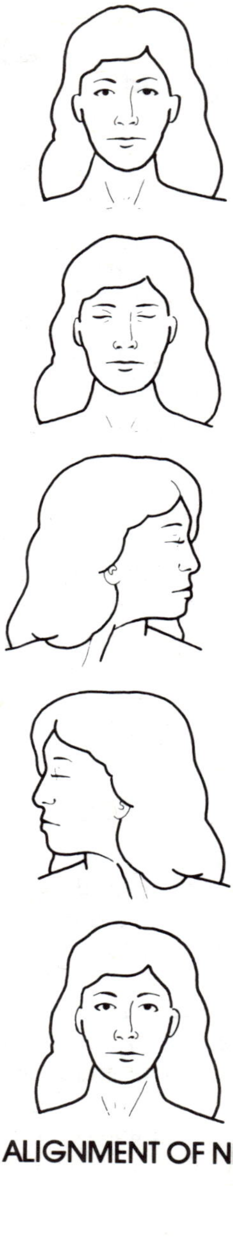

Figure 9-10

CHECKING ALIGNMENT OF NECK VERTEBRAE

In this standing position, other visual checks can be made. How straight is the head in relation to the rest of the body? Is the head turned or tilted to one side? Ideally, it should not be.

Also check the shoulders. Is one shoulder higher than the other? Is one more forward while the other tends to be held back? Another check of this part of the body is to see whether or not a person's arms extend the same distance from the shirt sleeves. Unless one arm is anatomically longer than other, disproportionate arm length can signal a spinal problem resulting from a misalignment or subluxation in the upper thoracic region. Quite simply, the shoulders are hanging tilted rather than straight on the spine. This can also be indicative of scoliosis.

Another relationship to consider is the one between the spinal column and the hips. Does one hip appear to be higher than the other? Is the hip twisted forward at all? A telltale sign is that when pants are worn, one pant leg is higher than the other. The pelvis should be held in a midway position, neither tucking under or protruding outward.

The natural curves of the spine should not be exaggerated, neither overly curved nor flattened. Another good test for overall spinal alignment is to have the person bend forward to note the position of the spine. Is any part protruding? Is the musculature even on both sides? These standing visual checks will greatly aid in checking the spine for problems before they become serious.

A person can also be observed and tested in a supine (face-up) position. Have the subject stand at one end of a bed, sit down, then lie straight back, face-up, with feet extending an inch or two over the edge. This position allows you to check leg length. Most of us tend to flare our feet and ankles out slightly. If this is the case, merely grasp the feet lightly and rotate them back to center. Then look down between the ankles.

Is one leg longer than the other? If so, chances are that one side of the body is under greater stress than the other. Once the leg check is done, you can look across the person, viewing the top of the body. Doing this will enable you to detect even slight differences in the flaring of the legs and the height of the pelvis. Does the pelvis appear to be sticking up higher on one side than the other? Sighting up the symphosis pubis (crotch) directly between the legs, through the sternum and the middle of the skull, will show deviations from the midline. You should be able to draw an imaginary straight line from the middle of the skull through the sternum and the crotch. The head should be pointing straight up, with the nose directly in the middle. These procedures cover the basics of checking someone lying face-up.

Observing a person lying prone (face-down) allows you to check the relationship of the back muscles. You can detect bunching of the muscles and variations on the skin line. The sacrum, the bottom portion of the spine connected to the pelvis, can also be viewed in this position. Does it appear to be higher on one side than the other? You will also be able to detect the relation of the alignment between the torso and the legs and pelvis. You may notice a slight contraction of the muscles of one side of the back, attributable to muscular or spinal misalignment.

Now you are aware of the various types of motions of which your spine is capable and exercises designed to maintain spinal flexibility. Once you are armed with this basic understanding of spinal function and maintenance, the next step is to explore the spine's daily use and some common spinal problems.

10

DAILY USE AND PROBLEMS OF THE SPINE

"You must do the thing
you think you cannot do."

Eleanor Roosevelt

One of our greatest fears about back problems is losing the ability to function normally on a day to day basis. The daily use of the spine largely determines its condition. Abusive use and lack of proper maintenance leads to a predisposition towards spinal problems. After having discussed the normal functioning of the spine, let's examine what happens when something goes wrong.

PROBLEMS OF THE NECK AREA

Several abnormal spinal conditions or subluxation configurations are, unfortunately, quite common. One frequently occurring abnormal condition is the "military neck." This condition is usually the result of a completely flattened neck curve, a flattened mid-back curve, and an increased low back curve. As the neck curve diminishes, the development of a sideways curve becomes obvious. When viewed front to back, a very straight neck tends to develop a pronounced sideways curve. Instead of normal curvature from the side, the neck now appears straight (Figure 10-1).

This is, potentially, a very serious condition. The head is no longer balanced properly, causing weight to bear on the joints on one side and stretching those on the other. A military neck is often aided in returning to normal curvature through lying on rolled towels, thus promoting the molding of proper spinal curvature.

Other abnormal spinal configurations occur from a reverse curve in the neck, usually caused by an injury. This is a dangerous condition, often interfering with the flow of nerve impulses in the upper spinal cord. It also makes movement of the neck area quite painful. Auto collisions often cause these conditions, especially hyperextension of the cervical spine, a trauma-induced neck injury commonly known as whiplash.

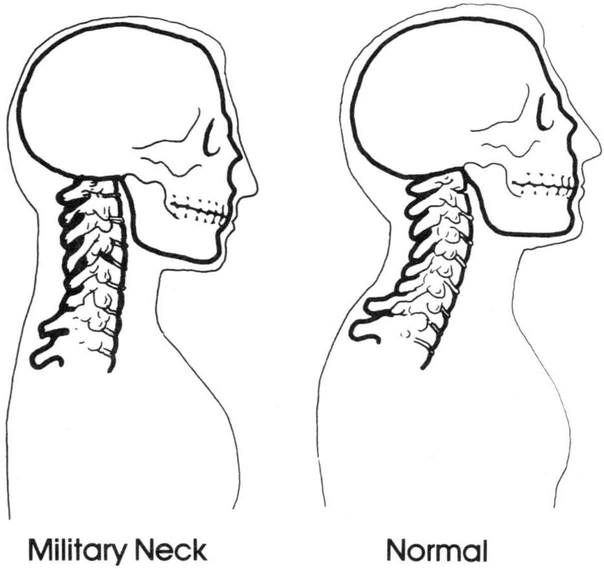

Figure 10-1 MILITARY NECK, SIDE VIEW

Though whiplash often causes immediate damage, its effects may not show up until later. After an automobile collision—days, weeks, even months later—many people experience such symptoms as headaches, dizziness, and loss of balance. These occur long after the cuts and bruises have healed.

Where do the symptoms originate? Often, they are the result of an improperly healed spine. Whiplash has the effect of literally tearing your head off your shoulders, displacing vertebrae in the process. This action stretches and tears muscles and ligaments that often never fully recover.

When the vertebrae are displaced through the force of a whiplash, damage can occur to the nerve roots as they exit the spinal cord. The result can be a lifetime of various disabilities, including paralysis. The situation is comparable to the tension strength of a spring. When you stretch a spring too far, it can never go back to its normal position. So it is with the ligaments that help reinforce the spinal column. Many whiplashes can be avoided, or at least the effects lessened by strengthening the muscles of the neck through spinal exercises. A good car seat with a properly fitted and functional headrest greatly reduces the chance of whiplash resulting from a vehicular collision.

It is vital that the spine be checked after any injury to ensure that there is no major damage to the structure. Don't confuse this with looking for broken bones, torn muscles, or ligaments. Most of the time they can be repaired and will heal adequately. Look to the condition and position of the spinal vertebrae and the discs which separate and cushion them.

Another common result of whiplash is a condition known as "stairstepping" of the discs and vertebrae. The angle of the vertebrae and discs is no longer in a curve; each one protrudes a little further than the one above or below, like stairs. If this condition goes unchecked, it becomes permanent and can lead to a lifetime of problems. If you doubt the damage whiplash can do, ask an insurance company how often whiplash injuries occur and how many people are still being treated five years later. Some must be treated for life. This is one more reason why spinal awareness is so important.

PROBLEMS OF THE MID-BACK

The thoracic spine has a normal curvature that runs in the opposite direction of the cervical curve above it and the lumbar curve below it. Too often, a person has too much curvature in the thoracic region. This condition, quite prominent in elderly people, is due either to a muscular weakness or, more commonly, to an alteration of the shape of the vertebrae.

With too much curvature abnormal vertebrae, viewed from the side, are no longer rectangular as they should be. Instead, they are wedge-shaped, narrower in the front than in the back. In the process of aging, a condition known as osteoporosis, a thinning of the calcium structure of the bone, often develops. As a result, the front portion of the bone collapses under the weight of the body, causing the shape of the vertebrae gradually to change from rectangular to wedge-shaped (Figure 10-2).

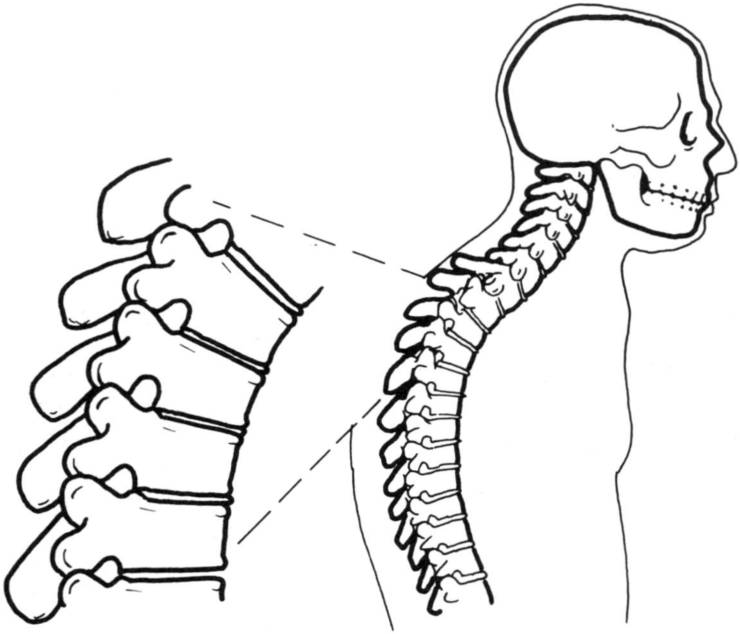

ABNORMAL CURVATURE OF THE THORACIC SPINE

Figure 10-2

Compression fractures, caused by falls or other impact injuries to the back, will also create an abnormal curve in the spine. This condition increases the curve in the upper portion of the neck. The lower portion of the neck begins to straighten out and increased curvature develops in the mid-back. In some instances, people develop a straight mid-back. These people have an almost regal bearing since they are relatively stiff in their appearance. When they turn their head, it doesn't appear to turn very far.

In this configuration, the mid-back curve is straightened. The neck curve is straightened or reversed, and the lower back curve increased. The lower back curve is relatively straight until you get to the last three vertebrae, which have a large curvature.

Scoliosis is an abnormal curvature of the spine which is visible in a front to back view of the spine. Scoliosis is often the result of one hip being higher than the other. Also, a sideways curvature develops in the middle portion of the spine, and one shoulder is generally higher than the other. By using the tests previously outlined in chapter nine, you can visually check another person for this condition (Figure 10-3).

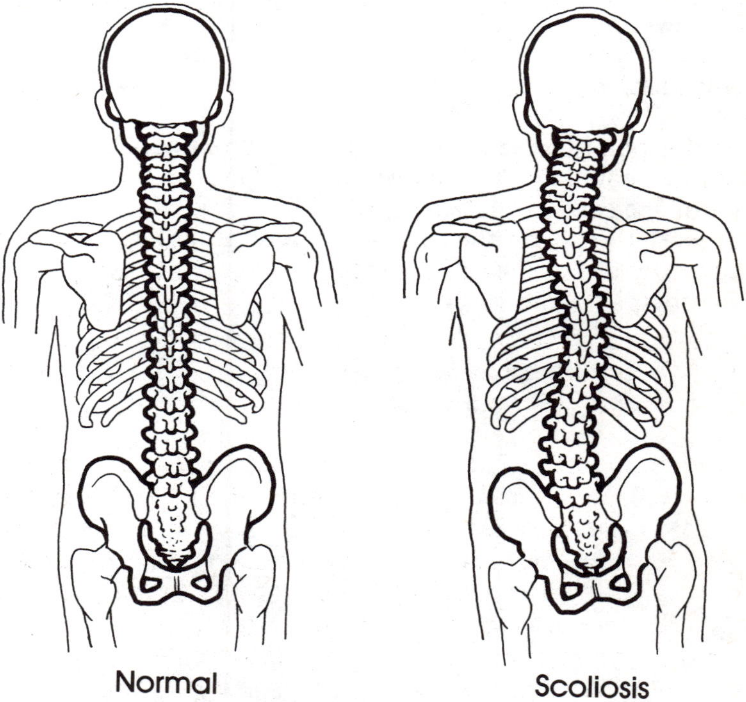

Figure 10-3 SCOLIOSIS OF THE SPINE

PROBLEMS OF THE LOWER BACK

In problems specifically related to the lower back, you are often dealing with either too much or too little curvature. When there is too much curvature in the lower back, the mid-back and neck curves are generally relatively normal. The excessive curve is compensated for primarily by the legs and the hips. The front part of the hips tends to come forward, resulting in more stress on the knees and leg muscles.

A diminished curve in the lower back results in a relatively straightened back continuing to the neck. People with this tendency walk very rigidly. The hips perform the motion ordinarily accomplished by the low back.

As previously mentioned, the spine has curves when viewed from the side but should appear straight when viewed from the front or back. It is critical to understand that when curvature is lost in one dimension (front to back) it is gained in another (side to side). If your spine were straight in both dimensions, like a broomstick, you would have practically no capacity for movement.

At this point let me draw an analogy. Years ago, cars had to be started manually. A crank was inserted into an opening in the front of the car to start the engine. The crank had a lever arm. This lever turned on the center of motion of the crank. This action provided the leverage needed to overcome the resistance of the engine (Figure 10-4).

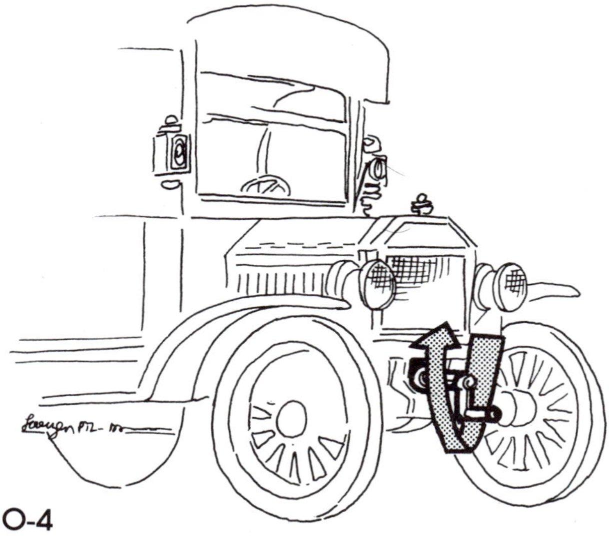

Figure 10-4

CRANKING ACTION OF A MODEL T AUTOMOBILE

What if the crank had no lever arm and simply protruded straight out from the engine? You would have to twist it, but you would have no leverage with which to work. It would be much harder to start the car. So it is with the spine. No curvature, no leverage. No leverage, no movement.

SLIPPED DISC — A MISNOMER

A common misconception regarding the spine has to do with the condition known as a "slipped disc." The term implies the disc has slipped out of place. Rarely does that happen (Cyriax 13). What often occurs is a rupturing of the disc due to improperly aligned vertebrae, trauma, or problems associated with posture, bending, or lifting.

Think of discs in terms of a peanut butter and jelly sandwich. If you squeeze the bread together, the peanut butter and jelly ooze out. When vertebrae are far enough out of position, they can push on the disc between them, causing the disc to rupture in the same way as the bread pushes on the peanut butter and jelly (Figure 10-5).

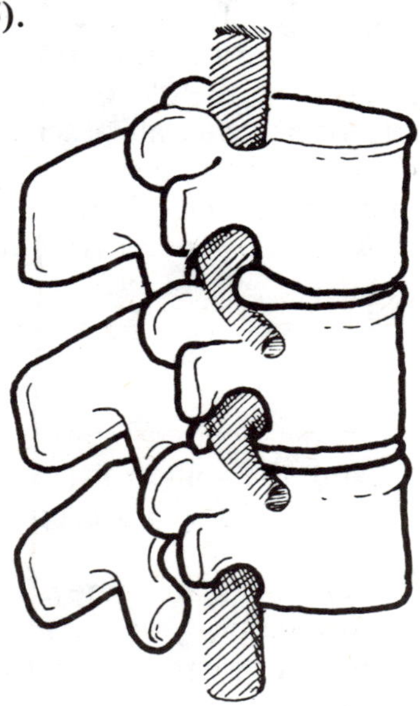

Figure 10-5

RUPTURED DISC

The cartilage composing discs are devoid of a direct blood supply. Since the healing mechanisms of the body depend on a direct blood supply, it is difficult for the discs to heal properly. Formation of scar tissue often results.

Sciatica is an example of a common disc related problem. This results from one or more discs pressing on the sacral nerves, the largest nerves of the body. Sacral nerves emerge from the lower part of the spine on either side of the hips and extend down the legs. Pain from this condition can be felt in the hips and lower back as well as radiating down the legs.

When surgery is recommended for a so-called slipped disc, the ruptured disc extending beyond the vertebrae is removed. That does not solve the problem if the cause is improperly aligned vertebrae. Vertebrae out of alignment cause unnecessary strain on the discs through improper weight distribution of the body on the spinal column. After the disc is cut through surgery, you may have a permanent reduction in mobility and use of the spine in that area, an example of a problem first getting out of hand, then being improperly treated (Cyriax 82 ff.). It only worsens with time.

Any surgery recommended for a back problem demands another opinion. Should the surgery not be successful, you may have to live with limitations for the rest of your life. Use surgery only as the last resort, after trying all other methods of treatment. You have the greatest control over improving your spine's condition through changing habits of posture and movement, exercise, and working with your doctor in following prescribed recommendations.

SLEEPING

In addition to preparing the spine for sleep, the position in which you sleep and the type of bed you sleep on has to be taken into consideration.

When you sleep on your back, the spine is in its most normal position: straight. Additionally, your diaphragm is not restricted, allowing you to breathe easier. There is no undue stress on your joints and muscles, and the body is in a natural relaxed position.

When sleeping on our side, we usually assume a fetal or similiar position. The head, however, may be improperly positioned. The skull should be 90 degrees to the plane of the shoulders. With the right size pillow, that is usually no problem. But with a pillow that is the wrong size, or during movement while asleep, your neck may not be in its best position. Sleeping on your side can also be hard on the shoulders. It tends to roll them forward and prolongs the healing of some shoulder injuries. The lower back gets support from the hips, however, so it should be fine (Figure 10-6). Though there are advantages to sleeping both on the back and the side, back care specialists agree that sleeping on the stomach is not advisable.

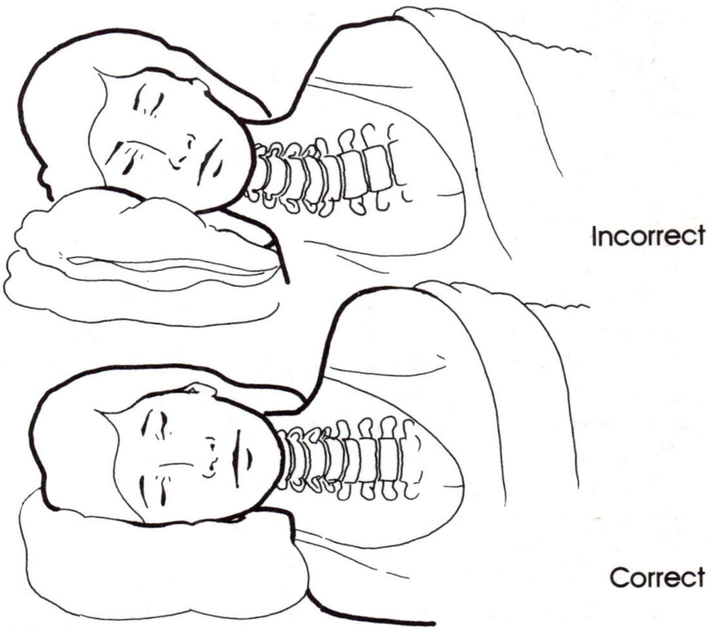

Figure 10-6

SLEEPING POSITIONS

Take a moment and turn your head as far as you can to one side. Think of holding it in that position for several hours. Sleeping on your stomach in this manner twists your neck severely. It is also hard to breathe in this position. Sleeping on your stomach can be a difficult practice to change, more so if you have been doing it a long time. Using the towels to relax the spine when going to bed can help you break the habit. Simply remove the towels after a few minutes and allow yourself to fall asleep on your back.

As you are lying on the towels, think about sleeping comfortably on your back. Visualize doing so. Visualize waking up in the morning on your back or side. Even when you take a nap this kind of preparation will help you sleep soundly in the correct position.

The other aspect of sleeping is the type and quality of your bed. The spine loves good firm, even support. It does not like sleeping on overly soft, lumpy surfaces such as an older, broken down mattress. Your bed should be strong enough to support your body comfortably and conform to its natural contours. Turning the mattress from head to foot and flipping it over periodically will preserve its shape and firmness for a longer period of time. Sleeping on a firm waterbed is also acceptable.

SITTING

Maintaining correct posture is also important when sitting. When somebody says, "Attention!" we straighten up. Good sitting posture is as simple as that. When you sit, sit up straight. Do not slouch or slide down in your chair as this puts more stress on your spine, which must work harder to hold you up.

Additionally, the spine begins to take on repeated abnormal configurations. If left unchecked, these configurations can lead to serious problems.

Crossing your legs while sitting can cut off your circulation and cause cramping. Avoid sitting with bulky objects such as a wallet in your back pocket. This forces one hip up higher than the other so that your pelvis and spine are not straight.

Rising from a sitting position can be done correctly and painlessly. It is best not to spring from the chair. First, move to the forward edge of the chair. Then spread your feet shoulder-width apart. Plant them under the forward edge of the chair. Lean the body forward slightly. Rise to a standing position, mainly using your leg muscles. Use your arms for support. Often we use our backs to rise from chairs and hurt them in the process. We have big thigh muscles for standing. Using them takes stress off the spine.

Getting in and out of a car is difficult for some people. If this is a problem for you, try this: Open the car door and sit down on the seat sideways with both feet outside flat on the ground. Once seated, lift the feet into the car and turn forward. When getting out of the car, swing your feet out and onto the ground. Then lift yourself up and out of the car.

RISING FROM A PRONE POSITION

Sometimes getting out of bed without pain can be facilitated by minimizing the stress on your back. To do this, lie on your side near the edge of the bed. While keeping the spine and legs in line, ease the feet forward off the mattress. Push upward with the hands and elbows, the legs and feet acting as a counterweight. Then use your hands to push your body upwards while slowly swinging the feet to the floor. By keeping your back straight, you will be in a sitting posture on the edge of the bed (Figure 10-7).

STANDING AND WALKING

How many of us have been shown how to walk correctly? As we grow up, the way we walk is often developed from imitating the walk of our parents and other role models. It is something acquired without much thought. How we walk says a lot about us and the condition of our spine. In theater, the way actors walk and carry themselves says a lot about the characters they are portraying. It is no different in day to day life.

Walking starts by standing properly. Good standing posture means evenly distributing your weight from your heels through the area of your arch or instep to the metatarsals or balls of your feet. People tend, however, to stand on their heels. This puts pressure on one-third of the foot instead of the weight being

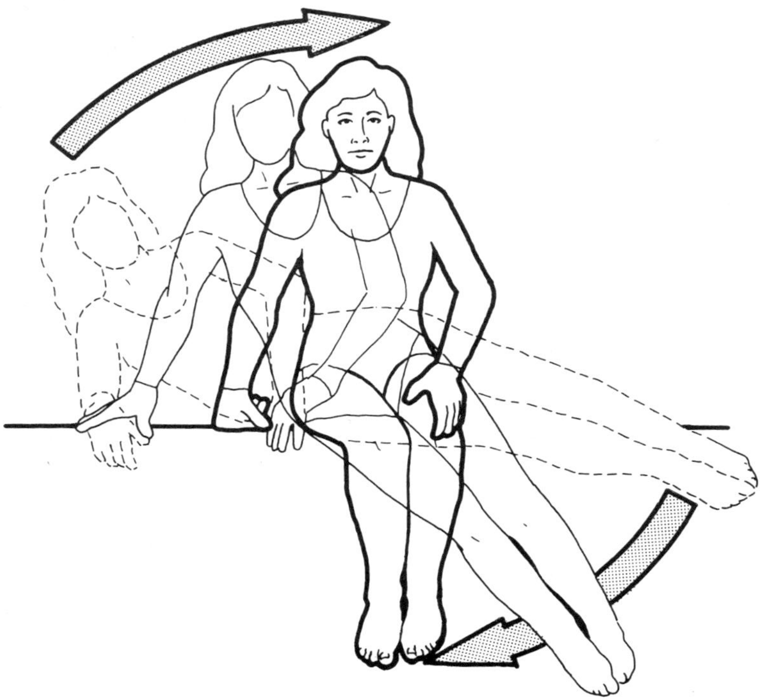

RISING FROM PRONE POSITION

Figure 10-7 Adapted from Cyriax, 1971

evenly distributed. The body weight should be centered evenly across the metatarsal (ball) of the foot. Many people walk on the inside or outside of their feet, which creates instability in the feet as well as not balancing the weight properly (Figure 10-8).

To walk properly, push off with one foot, landing first on the heel and then the center of the metatarsals of the other foot. Each leg alternates between a standing and a swinging phase. While the supporting leg pushes off, the other swings forward. When the swinging foot lands on the ground, the weight should be slightly ahead, about a half inch from the back of the heel. The arms should be relaxed and swinging. The hand that is swinging backwards almost grazes the hip as it passes. The arms are always swung opposite the leg movement. Right arm and left leg move forward; left arm and right leg move forward. By flexing your elbow slightly and increasing your arm swing, you can walk faster.

Looking straight ahead, walk with a sense of determination and purpose. Move from your center, which is an inch or so below your navel. Many of us walk from the shoulders with our bodies bent forward. Watch yourself walk in a store window or a mirror at home. This will help you to identify how you walk and correct any improper habits. Walking should be done in a fluid, rhythmic manner, neither too fast nor too slow. The body should act with coordination between the moving parts.

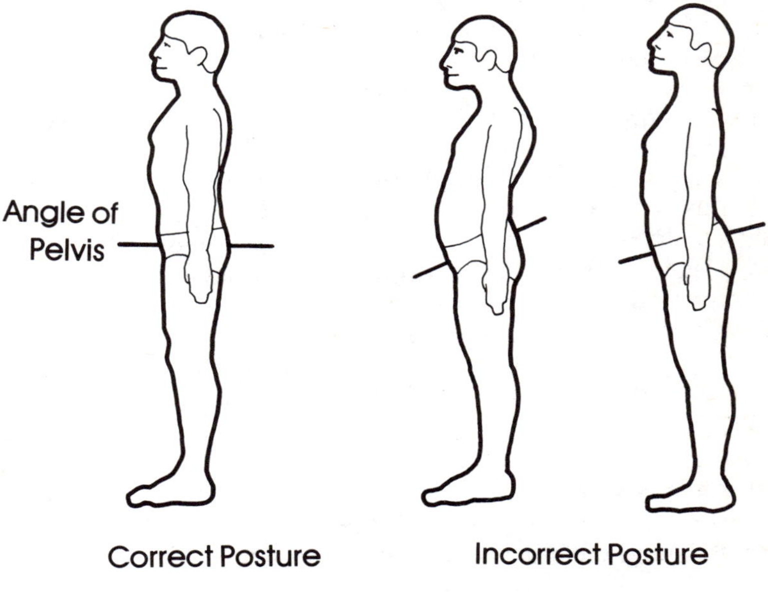

STANDING POSTURES

Figure 10-8

FOOTWEAR

Restrictive footwear and clothing can often hinder good spinal health, sometimes prohibiting the body's full range of motion. High-heeled shoes are an example, as they cause the pelvis to rotate forward. The visual effects of wearing high heels are well recognized. They definitely put an attractive sway in a lady's walk. They also increase the curve in the lower back. From that comes the back pain and muscle strains associated with having the back out of balance while trying to compensate for high heels all day. Wearing high-heeled shoes is considered a necessary part of a woman's wardrobe, yet doing so can be damaging to the health of the individual. Low-heeled footwear which keeps the body in a natural state of balance should be worn whenever possible (Figure 10-9).

Old shoes can also be unfavorable to your spine if overly worn on one side or the other. Shoes are an excellent indicator of how you distribute your body weight and how you walk. In the best circumstances, shoes should wear evenly. If they become overly worn on one side, (which could indicate a spinal problem), continued wear only promotes the problem. Spinal stress often results.

Although many people wear heel lifts, it's very important that such aids are used wisely and under the supervision of a qualified doctor. In some instances, a person may have an anatomically short leg. The heel lift, worn under the heel, acts as compensation. Heel lifts should be checked periodically to make sure their size remains correct.

LIFTING

Improper lifting can play havoc with your spine, especially when it involves bending over. A few rules of thumb will help you understand the best way to lift objects.

First, it is vital that your spine is warmed up before you do any lifting. Always warm up the spine through spinal twisting before doing ANY activity. Second, get as close as you can to the object you are picking up. Having something close to your body is much better than extending your arms too far. Third, lift with your legs, not your back. When you lift, bend the knees and squat down, not over. Maintain the proper curvature in your lower back at all times. Bending over removes the normal

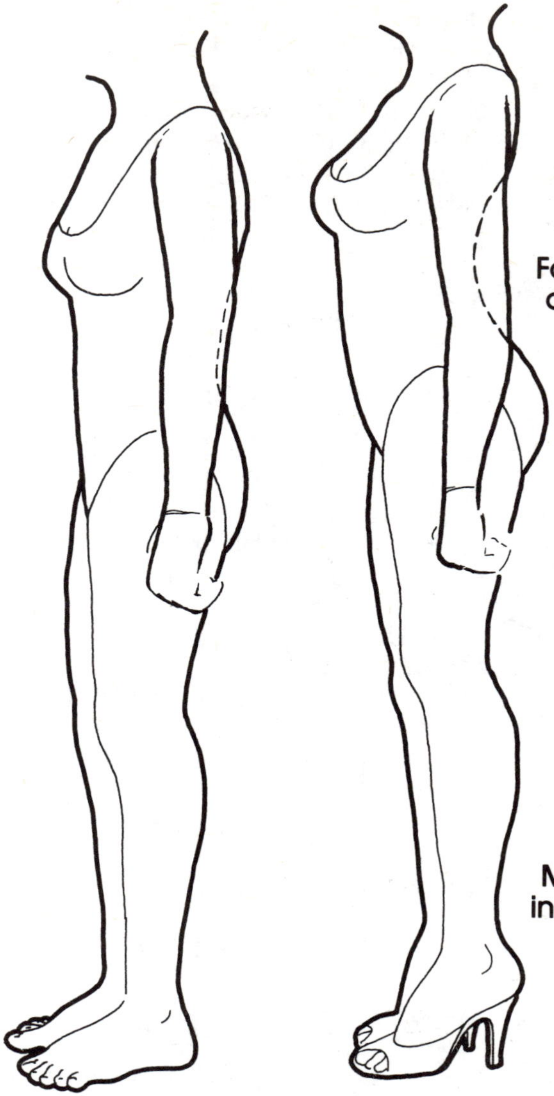

HIGH HEEL SHOES

Figure 10-9

curvature, eliminating leverage so the lower back ends up carrying the entire load itself. That's why we have thigh muscles. They should do the lifting, and the back should be the stabilizing force. Weight lifters wear a thick belt around their lower back in order to maintain proper curvature in their lumbar spine at all times. Using common sense when lifting can prevent many injuries, as well as the pain and suffering that accompanies them (Figure 10-10).

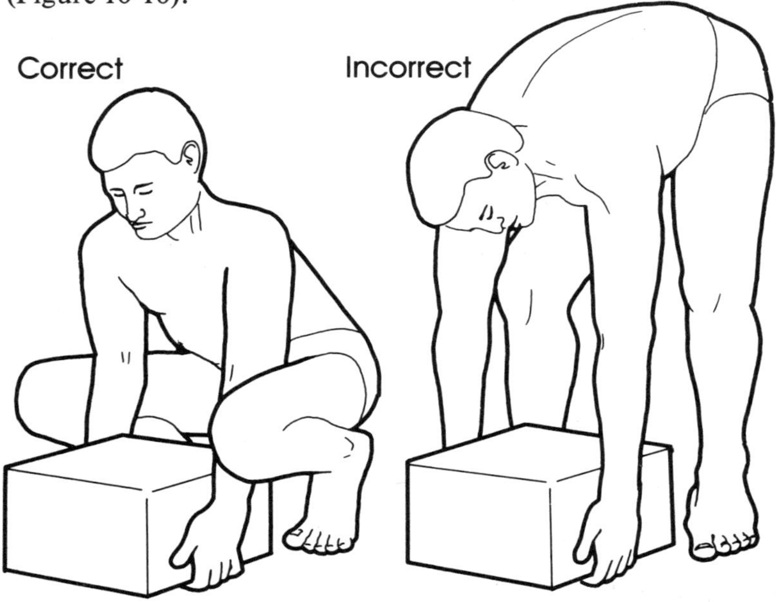

LIFTING POSTURES

Figure 10-10

DANGERS OF SELF-MANIPULATION

It is well documented that we have an epidemic of back problems in this country. Most of us will not go through life without having a back problem at one point or another (Rowe 1). In our efforts to correct these problems, many people resort to crude and dangerous methods in their attempts to relieve themselves of back pain and discomfort.

A common practice is to have somebody walk on your back. This is done to work out kinks, loosen up tight muscles, and get the person to relax. It is, however, quite dangerous, as it can be very harmful to the spinal column.

As mentioned previously, it is important NOT to put more force into the spinal column than it can resist on its own. Walking on a person's back can put more force into the spinal column than it can handle.

Another similar problem is associated with a person torquing the neck or lower back and "cracking" it. Again, this is done to eliminate stress and tension, making it easier to move the spine comfortably. This is also a very dangerous practice. I don't recommend doing it.

If you have a stiff spinal column, discomfort or tension in your back, chances are your spine is not capable of functioning throughout a normal range of motion. That being the case, try the exercises I have suggested for a month or two, using some massage in conjunction with them. If after a month or so, your problems persist, you probably have subluxations or other associated problems in your spinal column that require professional care.

As another form of compensation for spinal misalignment, many of us make gestures such as shrugging our shoulders, moving our head to one side, arching our back, and so on. After a while we begin to associate these methods of posturing with certain people and come to think of their movement as part of their personality and characteristics.

What they are subconsciously doing is compensating for the position and condition of their spinal column. Another axiom is that the body has a built-in or innate function that provides for the eyes to always look straight ahead, being level in relation to the ground. Therefore, the body often must contort itself to enable the eyes to look always straight ahead while remaining upright in resistance to gravity. In the process, certain areas of a misaligned spinal column are constantly under greater stress. Consequently, we move our bodies in various configurations as a way of compensation. This is where the twisting exercises and regularly putting the spine through a full range of motion will help the body to realign itself. As a result, you will function with greater ease.

Spinal self-awareness (being aware of how your spine is used on a daily basis) is vital because the spine is involved in virtually all of life's activities. Most of us are not interested, of course, in becoming experts in anatomy and physiology. But when armed with the information this book covers regarding the spine and its use and care in daily life, you can make a measurable and immediate impact on your health and the quality of your life.

11

MASSAGE: THE ART OF TOUCHING

"The greatest discovery of any generation is that human beings can alter their lives by altering their attitudes of mind."

Albert Schweitzer

Massage, rubbing, or stroking of a person's body by hand is an effective way of helping another person's spine relieve stress and maintain proper alignment. After you have used the visual tests previously described, massage can provide an excellent adjunct to care of the spine.

For centuries, many cultures have practiced the art of massage. It is much like animals preening one another. As a form of touching, massage has many benefits. Touching fulfills basic human needs. It provides enjoyment, satisfaction, and a sense of acceptance or belonging. Health care practitioners are increasingly realizing the importance of touching. Physical contact through the hands provides communication between individuals in a unique, wordless way. Few of us ever turn down a good back rub. Massage is not only enjoyable, it also has theraputic value. It helps the body rid itself of waste products, increases flexibility, and reduces stress. Massage is a form of communication from which we can all benefit.

Unfortunately, massage suffers from several negative sexual connotations which society attaches to it. People confuse touching with sexuality or having sex. Their belief is that you can't have one without the other. Today, however, the use of massage is increasing as a theraputic remedy in both sports medicine and for the treatment of routine injuries.

Relaxation, best facilitated through proper breathing, allows for the full benefit of massage. During massage you experience your body in a different way. Consciously controlling your breathing allows you to communicate with your body. It helps put you in a receptive physical state. Proper breathing helps you better eliminate stress and assist the communication between you and the person administering the massage.

There are many effective massage techniques. All have their place. Deep or heavy (painful) massage is used for the treatment of injuries or to remove large blockages of scar tissue, often the result of the healing of old injuries. The softer massage techniques are used to improve muscle tone, relaxation, flexibility, and blood circulation.

Massaging along muscle tissue lines likewise increases flexibility, circulation, and removal of toxins. Swedish massage is likely to be the most familiar to people, whereby the flat of the hand is used in a smooth or kneading movement. Other forms of massage, such as accupressure and shiatsu, incorporate specific points, such as finger tips, knuckles, and elbows to remove blockages and adhesions.

In his book, *Massage Techniques,* D. Baloti Lawrence explains some of the therapeutic aspects of massage:

> Massage is not a panacea and must be used correctly. The effective practice of massage depends on a knowledge of anatomy, physiology, physical and emotional development, and various massage techniques. The condition of the person must be properly assessed so that it can be determined if massage will be beneficial.... Most people can give an emotionally soothing massage simply by applying a caring touch. However, in order to bring about changes within the body, thorough knowledge and skill are required.... Massage can help keep the body's various systems in a state of free-flowing health [54,55].

Massage helps to maintain the proper alignment of the spine and body through relaxing the back muscles and relieving tension. We accumulate tremendous amounts of stress in daily life, and it is imperative that we rid ourselves of it from time to time.

Being aware of what a person is feeling at that moment and helping him or her to relax are the first steps in preparing to give a massage. Let the expression of the other person's body (tension, stress, fatigue, anger, etc.) direct you. A sense of touch is as important as technique. It's that special sense which allows you to locate another person's areas of pain and stress. Because we are all unique, each situation calls for a careful selection of the techniques employed. There are guidelines to follow, but massage is not automatically done the same way every time.

Massage is best performed in a warm and relaxing environment. If a hard or painful technique is necessary, it is best to start with a softer touch and then increase the intensity. This prepares the body much the same as warming up prior to exercise. Otherwise, the body's defense system senses an invasion, becomes tense, and positive results are difficult to achieve.

A general procedure for massage is to start with the head and work down the body. The person may lie face up or down on a massage table or other fairly firm surface.

First feel the head, neck, and then the shoulders, being aware of tension, tight muscles, or pain. With the thumbs almost touching each other in the area of the fifth cervical vertebra, begin to feel the trapezius or upper neck muscles. Feel the relationship of the head to the rest of the body. Make sure that the neck and head become relaxed. Then gently feel under the skull line, using the tips of your fingers and thumbs. Starting very slowly at first, put the head through each of its three ranges of motion—side to side, up and down, ear to shoulder. Then combine the motions in a fluid manner, never going past the range of normal motion the person's neck is capable of at that time.

Use the tips of your fingers to gently massage the major muscles along the neck. Next, work the area of the trapezius and shoulders. Start by using overall motions and then become more specific. Slowly work any areas of pain or tenderness. Using this method, you can follow all the way down the spine. Always maintain contact with the body while you are massaging. Momentary loss of contact is similar to being disconnected on the phone.

After the spine and supportive structures, the feet are another area of importance in massage. Many of us love having our feet rubbed, especially after being on them all day. Start by touching softly, then working to release tension by separately working on the toes, arches, ankles, insteps, and so on. Put the foot through a full range of motion, including spreading the toes apart and moving them back and forth and up and down. Fortunately, the feet are a part of the body we can massage ourselves.

After the feet, massage the knees, elbows, and hands. Knees greatly benefit from massage. The knee joint is often under stress, especially through athletics. The knee is a hinge joint with little side to side capability. Unfortunately, athletics often subject the knees to this side to side motion. In fact, this occurs even in day to day life such as when we are walking. Many people walk with their weight placed too far forward, stressing the knees rather than utilizing the large thigh muscles which are meant to carry the weight. Flexing the leg puts the knee through a full range of motion. Moving the kneecap around slightly, plus lightly massaging any tender areas, can help bring relief.

Massaging areas of the body that will be in particular use prior to stressful activity—sports, for example—is quite helpful. This prepares these areas of the body for the forces they will inevitably encounter. Likewise, massaging a part of your body that is injured can speed up the recovery process. Rather than avoiding the area of discomfort, you are addressing it directly, focusing your body's healing powers as well as your own mind on it.

Massage is a valid form of preventive health care. It does wonders for maintaining the body and working out stress and discomfort before they become serious problems. It also better helps you to facilitate the relationship you have with your body.

12

PHYSICAL EXERCISE: A MIND AND BODY EXPERIENCE

"We spend our health in search of wealth,
we sweat, we toil, we slave.
Then spend our wealth in search of health,
and all we get's the grave."

Anonymous

Physical exercise is both a mental and physical activity. It involves the shape and size of your body as well as what you think of it.

Our bodies reflect our personalities. They reveal what we think of ourselves and our relationship with the world around us. The way we walk and carry ourselves, our mannerisms and style of movement all tell a lot about us.

Physical exercise is a means of relating to your body and allowing you to participate in life. When you haven't exercised for awhile, you lose your ability to function at your best. The body was designed for activity and longs for regular and extensive use.

Exercise is a must for anyone desiring an energized and productive life. It promotes an overall feeling of well-being that comes from having stamina of the heart and lungs, good flexibility of the joints, and the ability to invigorate the body through exerting a reasonable amount of energy. Exercise promotes a feeling of mental and physical vigor.

EXERCISING AND LIFE'S ACTIVITIES

A hundred years ago, many people performed physical labor, their bodies actively involved in what they did for a living. But physical labor is no longer a regular part of life for many people. Because of the automobile, the development of automation in the work place, and labor saving devices at home, our bodies aren't being utilized as they once were. Physical exercise is no longer a necessity. But for the sake of maintaining health, effort must be made to introduce and incorporate physical exercise into our daily routine. People generally exercise for physical appearance, self-respect, discipline, development, and for self-preservation.

Physical exercise can require a special routine and environment, such as working out at a club or health spa. But maintaining such a program on a regular basis can be difficult. We have careers, families, and other obligations that take our time. There are also times when we simply don't feel like going to the club or gym. So rather than being a natural and pleasant experience, getting physical exercise instead becomes a chore. We have to work at it.

These challenges are compounded by the fact that few of us have a good understanding of how our bodies operate. We understand finance, the sciences, and art, but have little working knowledge of the living mechanism (our bodies) that makes everything else possible.

THE WEEKEND WARRIOR

If one hasn't exercised for a long time, the body requires time to get used to doing so again. We call this "getting back into shape." But we see ads for the perfect, slim, sexy body, seemingly obtainable in a matter of weeks. Practical wisdom goes out the door and we become ripe for injuries. Can you blame someone for not wanting to exercise after getting hurt by starting an overly strenuous exercise program? At that point, the negatives outweigh the positives.

How many times have you had little or no activity throughout the week and then become a weekend warrior? No wonder we hate Mondays. After doing nothing all week, we over exercise and thus abuse ourselves on the weekend. We then have to put up with discomfort the following week. This is both mentally and physically dangerous. Surprising the body with a twenty mile hike or a day of skiing after weeks of inactivity is inviting trouble. The body is not prepared for the amount of effort it must expend and cannot smoothly and effectively handle the exertion.

Giving your body a good workout and brutilizing it are two different things. The number of injuries sustained by weekend warriors keeps a lot of doctors busy Monday through Friday. Many of these injuries also come back to haunt us when they are not treated or improperly treated in the first place. When tempted to become a weekend warrior, take a moment to consider that you may be setting yourself up for injury you will regret for years to come. This is the common sense approach to health.

THE KEY TO EXERCISE: BECOMING A PART OF YOUR LIFESTYLE

Exercise must be slowly and easily integrated into your lifestyle. If it isn't, you won't keep at it for long. Many of us function like we're on a roller coaster. We work out for a month, stop for a month, work out again for a month or two, stop again for six months. This on again, off again style develops into a lifelong pattern.

How many of us make a diet or exercise program part of our New Year's resolutions? We usually last about six weeks, until Valentine's day. Then in the spring, we decide to get into shape for summer. Summer comes and we never quite made it. Next comes fall. We figure with the holidays coming with their usual onslaught of goodies, why bother? We go through this cycle year after year. Isn't the ride getting old by now? Do you ever wonder if there is a better way? The key is to make exercise part of your lifestyle. Otherwise it will never become continuous and permanent.

Some mental preparation must take place to coincide with the physical activity. An honest evaluation of ourselves is a must. First, we must remove our own self-inflicted guilt that is a result of our behaviors. Guilt and bad feelings are detrimental to our growth and progress. How often do we say, "Well, I didn't work out tonight and I'll probably miss tommorrow. Why bother?" This kind of rhetoric must be eliminated.

The hardest aspect of exercise is not the time spent working out. It's the first time you don't work out. That's when you start playing mental games. It is easy to say that since you missed yesterday, you'll probably miss today. Whatever amount of good work you've already done then goes down the drain.

Starting and stopping programs does nothing beneficial for you and just makes the health clubs rich. Once you've paid the money and the initial excitement of joining a club wears off, it's just you by yourself. The club is busy selling a membership to somebody else. As in a relationship, getting past the romance and into day to day life claims many casualties.

Don't berate yourself and mentally crumble everytime you go off your diet or exercise program. Nobody is perfect. We all fall short. Too often we forget that and expect ourselves to be perfect.

Instead, remind yourself that you are human and therefore shouldn't be expected to follow a rigid, unyielding program all the time. Rather, after having missed a day, acknowledge that you are human and that you will fall short occasionally. Then forget about it and start again the next day. Don't let missing a day of exercise become the rationale for not continuing along with your program.

Give yourself credit for what good you have done, not criticism for where you fall short. Emphasizing your shortcomings gives you license to continue falling short. You are telling yourself that you are not O.K. and to prove it, you act out your shortcomings over and over again. Concentrate on maintaining your program for the long term. Continue to persist in spite of minor delays.

Most of us don't like doing what we don't do well. If you don't think you're good at exercising, you simply have a mental obstacle to overcome. Unless you remove it, you will come up against this mental barrier every time you do something physical. Mental blocks prevent us from taking action, having new experiences, and growing.

Beware! Don't let advertisements dictate what you should look like and what you should be doing to stay in shape. Advertisements promote products and services for the purpose of making money. They control us by making us want to be something we're not. The image they try to sell us is not real. The perfect looking body is the ultimate advertising illusion. In those fleeting moments when reality sets in, you realize what is happening. The desire to exercise should be your own personal choice, not because somebody has sold you a bill of goods.

Some people are naturally more physically active than others. If you are one of those persons, consider yourself lucky. You're that much further ahead. Many other people, though, have a problem of not liking their bodies. Rather than being a harmonious expression of their mental and physical selves, they feel their body is a prison in which they are doomed to dwell. Finding enjoyment in exercise can help solve this problem.

ENJOYING EXERCISE

Physical exercise should be fun. Many of us forget that. We have the impression that exercise is hard work and if you enjoy it for some reason, you are doing it wrong. The fact is, exercise or any physical activity that is fun is what you are more likely to do over a longer period of time. Why not build a program around what you like to do? It's better than trying to make yourself do penance. The trick is to get the most results for the amount of time and effort spent.

To be effective and provide lasting benefits, physical exercise must become an enjoyable part of your lifestyle, like taking a shower, shopping, or going to the movies. That, above all else, is the best kind of exercise. If exercise doesn't fit into your lifestyle, you won't stay with it very long.

Many people say that the biggest obstacle to exercising is lack of time. Although that may be true to some extent, it is also a self-limiting concept. Not having the time is a socially acceptable reason we often use as an excuse. Believing you don't have the time will stop you from doing anything before you ever get started.

Having time is an obvious necessity and makes planning essential. You have to realize honestly and objectively where you spend your time. Look at where time could be spent on exercise. Exercise is that portion of daily physical activity that is planned, structured, repetitive, and has a sense of purpose in that an objective is the improvement or maintenance of physical fitness (Nieman 33).

If you cannot take time to drive to the gym and work out regularly, look at alternative ways to integrate exercise into your lifestyle. Exercise equipment and programs such as on video tapes are becoming more available for home use.

Some people, however, are more accountable because of the peer pressure and social contact provided by the club or gym. As a result, they may do more there than at home. Ask yourself what would be the ideal situation for you. It is essential that you maximize your time to get the fullest possible benefit from what you are doing. This is doubly true if you spend only two hours or less a week in structured physical activity.

Once the issue of time and what to do with it is handled, repetition is the next key word. The best exercise is any physical activity you can and will do often. This goes the furthest towards keeping your body in shape. Exercise is like faith. It must be practiced regularly. Only then are the benefits of exercise cumulative.

An important point to remember about exercise is that some exercise is better than none at all. Those who spend a lot of time on their bodies will get the most benefits. If you are going to spend only a minimal amount of time exercising, however, you must at least make it effective. This means exercising intelligently. How you exercise, how much, and how consistent you are counts significantly.

Integrating exercise into your lifestyle takes effort, commitment, and creative thinking. Look at the areas of your life which can help you get more exercise. For example, most of us go to the store fairly regularly. Our tendency is to park as close as possible. We don't want to walk any farther than is necessary. Is this due to laziness or conditioning? Are we afraid to park farther away and walk a little bit? We even spend a minute or two driving around the parking lot looking for the closest space to the entrance. What if you were to park at the other side of the parking lot? What does it take to walk the extra distance to the store, a minute or so? You spend that much time driving around, looking for a closer parking space.

Walking across the parking lot will not put you in world-class shape. It will, however, give you a little extra exercise. Your body will appreciate that more than driving around unnecessarily. In addition, try incorporating walking or bicycling instead of always taking your car.

The same holds true for stairs. Most buildings with two or more floors often have both an elevator and stairs. But doesn't almost everyone take the elevator? Stairs offer another everyday opportunity to give your body some activity. Using stairs will exercise your legs, lungs, and cardio-vascular system. Changing personal habits provides opportunity for the body to experience physical activity. Making these changes fun and enjoyable rather than drudgery is a mature and effective approach.

THE MECHANICS OF EXERCISE

This brings us to the mechanics of why one physically exercises and what constitutes a good exercise program. Understanding these concepts is a matter of learning a few basics about how the body operates and what it needs to stay in shape.

What is physical exercise? It is putting your body through a structured range of activity. There are three aspects in which exercise can produce benefits: physical flexibility, cardio-vascular development, and muscular strength and endurance.

A good exercise program develops and maintains physical flexibility. Like the spine, the body must be put through a full range of motion on a regular basis. This ensures the spine's continued usefulness and therefore, your overall ability to move. In that respect, being flexible allows you to better physically function in your life.

Cardio-vascular development takes place when the body is in action at a controlled level for twenty minutes or longer. You increase the activity until the heart is operating at about three quarters of its maximum capacity. Your lungs also get a good workout. Extending your heart and lungs to this capacity puts them through a full range of use.

If you haven't exerted your heart and lungs in a while and then use them strenuously, you will notice how fast you tire. The heart and lungs cannot keep up. They have gotten out of condition.

Exercise also develops strength, especially in the tendons and muscles of the body. After warm-up and some cardio-vascular activity, the body is ready for strength building. Progressive resistance to the muscles, such as lifting weights, is an excellent way to build strength and increase muscle size.

It is helpful to understand why we need physical exercise. Exercise affects the body in three ways: structurally, chemically, and emotionally. Structurally, exercise builds strength, increases flexibility, and helps to keep the joints and organs (lungs and heart) working properly. Chemically, exercise uses up energy derived from the food we eat. Without doing this, the energy would be stored as fat, making us larger and larger all the time. Cleansing of the body is accomplished through sweating and breathing.

Emotionally, physical exercise lightens your mood and helps to relieve depression. Exercise helps you to gain a positive feeling of control of your body. More importantly, it helps to integrate your mind and body. We live in our bodies. How can we avoid having a relationship with them? Having a good relationship between the mind and body is a truth about health.

TYPES OF EXERCISE

A variety of exercises in which to participate are available today. The key is finding ones that meet your individual needs and capabilities. Exercises fall into four basic categories: isometric, isotonic, anaerobic, and aerobic.

Isometric exercise is designed to contract muscles without producing movement. They act to increase muscle size and strength but have little benefit to offer the heart or lungs. In isometrics, muscles work equally against each other or an immovable object. An example would be pushing against the opposite sides of a doorway or doing a pushup where you keep the body in a constantly lowered position. This form of exercise is highly advantageous for bedridden patients by preventing atrophy of the muscles and helping them develop strength.

Isotonic exercise is similar to isometrics in that it works primarily on the muscles. The major difference is that when the muscles are contracted, movement is produced. Weightlifting is a good example of isotonic exercise. Isotonics minimizes cardiovascular development and should therefore not be exclusively used when achieving overall body conditioning.

Anaerobics are exercises of high intensity done for very short periods of time. An example would be swimming underwater or sprinting a hundred yard dash. Exercises of this nature derive energy from the body's glycogen (sugar) reserves since short, high intensity energy requirements need a rapid breakdown of glycogen. Anaerobics are used by some athletes, but caution must be used by the average person. You should not demand more from your body than it is capable of safely giving or has been trained for.

Aerobics is a commonly practiced form of exercise that increases the body's ability to take in oxygen, a conditioning process which in time develops stamina and endurance. The key to aerobic exercise is moderate intensity of long duration. The amount of time spent is the essence of it. The intensity level must be kept low enough so you can sustain yourself for at least twenty minutes. Twenty minutes to a half hour three times a week is an excellent starting point. A good body conditioning program should include both aerobic and isotonic activity.

Make an honest evaluation of how much time you will spend exercising. That is the basis for a realistic approach. Build a program that will sustain you throughout your life. When life is devoid of physical activity for a long time, the brain loses its awareness and frame of reference for that experience. The body will no longer be as adept at performing.

As children, most of us were full of energy and very active. We spent the majority of our time developing our bodies. We learned what they could do and how to use them. We became involved in sports or other structured activity in high school and perhaps college. But what happened when we stepped out into the adult world? How does exercise fit into our daily routine? Is it harder to find opportunities for frequent physical activity? When there are no means or reasons to stay in good physical shape, do we tend to let our bodies go?

You must have a purpose in mind to sustain physical exercise on a regular basis. Since time is often limited, you have to make it count. Exercise must be important enough to you that you will do it for yourself.

EXERCISE AND DAILY LIFE

Physical exercise can be integrated into your daily life, beginning with the start of your day. At that time, twisting your spine is the most important exercise to do first since it prepares your spine and therefore your body for activity. If you have some time and motivation after twisting your spine, work in ten minutes or so of exercise. It's great to help get you going in the morning, especially if you don't do anything else energetic throughout the day.

Forget the chic outfits and all the sweating. Do a little warm-up to get your heart pumping. Jumping rope is great for that. How about doing a few pushups, muscle toning, or an aerobic activity? Play your favorite music while you exercise. All of this costs nothing extra. It can be done in the privacy of your own home. Exercise like this prepares you mentally and physically for the day.

Take the opportunity to credit yourself for having done something for yourself. Early morning exercise minimizes your chances of injuring yourself, especially your back. You will have warmed up your body and have better prepared it physically for the day. Just doing that is a major accomplishment.

How many people injure themselves doing seemingly safe things? Every day people are hurt getting in and out of bed, the shower, the car, even taking out the garbage. Their bodies probably were not ready for the activity. Early morning activity may also reduce the need for coffee, the great American caffeine fix.

If it is possible, exercise again after work or at another time of the day. A few minutes is better than none at all. And remember to have fun!

As children most of us did enjoyable things that also provided physical exercise. These activities included swimming, biking, running, walking, just being outside and playing. Activities that are fun increase your chances of doing them on a regular basis. Think also of doing different things to provide variety. Even seasoned athletes will tell you they get bored with the same exercise routine. Be creative. People get injured when exercise becomes a drudgery. They really don't want to do it, but they force themselves. They are mentally resisting it, becoming more apt to cause injury to themselves.

Sometimes we don't fully warm up the body. We rush through the motions of exercise just to get finished. Results are better received when you focus on what you are doing. Exercise is no different than anything else. They know that it is better to stop and go home than risk injury by forcing themselves. Not only must you focus your attention during exercise, but attention must also be placed on developing a plan that you can follow and will last over the long term.

SET GOALS AND DEVELOP A PLAN

Health, like life, works best when you have a plan. Writing down goals clarifies what and why you are doing something. Think first, then act.

Few things are more powerful than having a plan to take you where you want to go in life. It focuses the mind, helping to create harmony in your life. Both the mind and body are working together for the common good. The reasons need only be your own.

Goals are what we want to accomplish in life. They are the purpose for getting out of bed in the morning. All of life's goals, whether physical or financial, family or spiritual, are beneficial when you consciously devote time to them on a regular basis.

What counts is clarity of purpose, which relates to the mental aspect of health. Putting your brain and body together maximizes both your time and results. Have your goals on paper and review them daily. The best times are the first thing in the morning, to give you focus throughout the day, and the last thing at night, to let your mind refine them while you sleep.

There are two important things to remember about goals. First, identify your destination. Second, have specific action steps to get you there. Four aspects to remember when working toward one's health goals are the following:

First, be oriented to your goals. They must be real to you, providing concrete benefits in your mind that you fully comprehend and want to achieve. Don't set them so high that they are unattainable.

Second, innovation and creativity are vital. Whether designing a way to exercise your biceps or losing a few extra pounds, the methods used to achieve your goals should be interesting and have variety.

Third, utilize constructive self-criticism. If we acknowledge where we fall short and move on, we advance more rapidly. Most of the time, everyone else can already see our shortcomings. Eliminating our shortcomings takes discipline on a daily basis.

Fourth, be personally accountable. In the end, you live with the results you create. Having goals and objectives allows you to make the right decisions today, providing you with the desired results tommorrow.

13

INTEGRATING YOUR INNATE INTELLIGENCE AND PHYSICAL BODY

"You, the individual, can do more
for your own health and well being
than any doctor, any hospital,
any drug, any exotic medical device."

Joseph Califano

Former U.S. Secretary of
Health, Education, and Welfare

FITNESS VERSUS HEALTH

Knowing why you exercise means understanding the difference between fitness and health. Fitness is our ability to perform physically. Health integrates both the inner and outer self as a whole being. It includes your habits and your physical performance. A lot of people are confused about this. They hear about people who are quite physically active (fit) dying of heart attacks (health). No account for the condition of their spine is ever made. What about their diet and condition of their internal organs? What about other habits, stress, and genetic factors that affected their health.

Fitness is only part of the total picture, though it is a very necessary part. Fitness can be defined in six major ways. First, it means endurance. This is work or exercise that lasts a long period of time. It primarily involves lung capacity and heart strength.

Second, fitness is flexibility level. Your suppleness allows you to bend without breaking.

Third, fitness is balance, how well centered you are, meaning how well your body keeps its state of balance while functioning.

Fourth, fitness is strength, that is, how strong you are and the condition of your musculature.

Fifth, fitness is speed, how fast you are capable of performing. Speed combined with strength results in power, desirable for athletics.

Sixth, fitness is coordination, how well the various parts of your body work together.

USING YOUR MIND TO BENEFIT YOUR BODY

Creative visualization and meditation are important techniques for helping our bodies. They help put the mind to work for the benefit of the body. Many bodybuilders practice visualization, imagining their muscles growing bigger as a result of lifting weights. In effect, they are channeling their energy to the muscles being worked.

Through meditation, creative visualization can be taken a step further by combining it with your goals. Meditation is one of the oldest forms of self-healing and methods of achieving spiritual balance. Virtually all cultures use it in one way or another. Meditation is an excellent form of self-therapy. Though there are endless ways to meditate, I speak of it in terms of relaxing the body, mentally visualizing your goals and your body, and assisting your body with its own healing and growth processes. The goal is to incorporate a realistic program into your daily life.

Soothing music is beneficial to meditation and relaxation, as it helps focus your attention on your inner self. Experiment a little to see what selections you like best. Especially appropriate for meditation are the soothing and relaxing sounds of classical and modern popular music. Recordings of natural sounds like those of birds, rainfall, and the sea shore can also be used.

Meditation in the morning prepares you mentally for the day's activites. At the same time, you can orient yourself to what your goals are and therefore remain on purpose throughout the day. You can make your own cassette tape and play it before or after the alarm goes off.

Use music at the start of the tape to make yourself aware of the world around you. Let the music slowly bring you to consciousness. Most of us are very receptive just before we fully awake. Then hear your goals being stated in a positive manner in your own voice and choice of words.

Goals can be physical, mental, social, financial, spiritual, or family oriented. State them in a positive manner in the present tense, as in the following example: "I see myself becoming thinner and more attractive as I exercise regularly. My body feels good and in condition. My life is becoming much more exciting.

I feel confident about myself and my appearance." These mental pictures should evoke a deep emotional response within you. When you picture your goal and get a strong feeling of its reality, your brain experiences the goal more fully. It is then more apt to work on it than when your goal is merely words.

While you listen, visualize yourself successfully achieving your goals. They will come about from the efforts you put forth. Your goals can be changed as often as necessary. The use of sounds and music is a soothing way to awaken yourself. Make the tape as long or short as you wish. Whatever the length of your tape, subtract its length of time from the time you must get out of bed. If you want to be up by 8:00 and the tape is 15 minutes long, it should start to play at 7:45. Allow yourself to adjust to the process. You'll soon enjoy it and find it very comforting.

EXERCISING PROPERLY

Exercise has many important and positive effects on the physical body. One is flexibility. Remember, "If you don't use it, you'll lose it." If you don't do much else in the way of physical activity, work at keeping your body as limber as possible. Naturally, this starts with your spinal column, the foundation of all movement.

Warm-up is the first necessary part of any exercise. It gets the body prepared for further activity. What is necessary is to get the heart rate up and increase the blood flow throughout your body. This can be done very simply. Examples would be simple calisthenics or riding a few minutes on a stationary bicycle. It is imperative that the body be warmed up in this manner before any stretching is done. Warming up the muscles prior to stretching makes them more flexible and better prepares the tendons and ligaments. The tendons and ligaments are often pulled when the body is forcefully exerted without a proper warm-up.

Stretching properly puts your joints, especially the spine, through a full range of motion. If you have ever studied yoga, you know the tremendous emphasis placed on limbering the spine and keeping it aligned properly. Yoga devotes a great deal of attention to the spine, and well it should. A few minutes of yoga each day not only stretches the body, but is also mentally and spiritually beneficial as well.

DEEP BREATHING

As a beneficial adjunct to a good warm-up, nothing beats deep breathing. Deep breathing in the morning prepares the lungs and respiratory systems for the day and puts them through their full range of use. Deep breathing works well while stretching because you are expanding your diaphragm. The diaphragm is composed of muscle and connective tissue that separates the thoracic and abdominal cavaties. The diaphragm pushes down on the abdomen during inhalation which provides greater room for the lungs to expand. Deep breathing also helps get rid of accumulated waste material in the lower portions of the lungs.

A major benefit of deep breathing and of exercise is that it purifies the body. It's one of the reasons you smell stronger after working out.

All night your lungs receive oxygen and get rid of carbon dioxide wastes from the blood. There is no better time to clean them out than when you rise in the morning. Many people are shallow breathers, using only a third or a half of their lung capacity. The rest goes unused. Unless you exercise and exert yourself, your lungs don't get adequate stimulation. They break down just like the rest of the body. "If you don't use it, you'll lose it" also applies to your lungs.

If you don't exercise much, deep breathing will give your lungs a little workout. It will provide you with more energy and help you awaken faster. Try a few minutes of stretching and deep breathing in the morning and whenever else you can.

OXYGEN: FOR HEALTH, ENERGY, & VITALITY

Oxygen is vital to our lives. It can be thought of as an invisible form of food. We can go without eating for days or even weeks. Without oxygen, we rarely survive for more than a few minutes. Oxygen is also the greatest of all purifiers. It is essential for a clean and pure blood stream.

Breathing is an innate, self-regulating process, like digestion and sleeping. It is natural to breathe correctly, and we do so from infancy. As we grow older, however, we tend to spend more time in a sitting position which can restrict breathing. Thus, we begin to depart from active and correct breathing.

Correct breathing is essential. Blood passes through the lungs to be purified and enriched by the oxygen we breathe. Lungs are spongy masses of porous tissue consisting of millions of tiny air cells called alveoli. These are surrounded by small blood vessels, called capillaries. Incoming oxygen passes through the delicate lining of the cells and mixes with the blood. The blood exchanges the oxygen for its waste products, known as carbon dioxide.

The heart takes the oxygenated blood from the lungs and sends it to the rest of the body. Through the capillaries the oxygen in the blood reaches the cells in the body. The carbon in the nutrients combines with the oxygen and creates waste, carbon dioxide.

This waste, caught up in the blood stream, is then sent back to the lungs, which expel the carbon dioxide and take in a fresh supply of oxygen. Sitting bent over or taking only shallow breaths results in not changing the air at the base of the lungs, where two-thirds of the lung capacity is located.

In such cases, the new blood, going back through the entire system, is now depleted in its supply of oxygen. It has less nourishment for the cells and has more difficulty eliminating the cells' waste products. Over the years this continual depletion contributes to a toxic body. Such a condition also points to the fact that a few basics, like proper breathing, are the real essentials to having a healthy life.

An obvious obstacle to good breathing is living and working in rooms without fresh air. Stagnant air, containing little oxygen, makes breathing difficult. It's important to have fresh air in our homes and at work. Besides the lungs, each muscle has different functions and tasks to perform. One set of muscles, the abdominal (stomach) muscles, is very important yet often overlooked.

EXERCISING THE ABDOMINAL MUSCLES

Abdominal or stomach muscles provide forward stabilization of the spinal column, keeping us properly balanced in an upright position.

The body normally stores fat around the midsection, some of which is designed to insulate and protect vital organs. But lifestyle factors, such as a poor diet and lack of exercise, result in people accumulating too much fat in this area. In our society, it has become commonplace to see men develop a "pot belly" as they get older. Over a period of time the effectiveness of the stomach muscles is diminished.

An oversized stomach results in forwarding our center of gravity. More stress is placed on the lower back muscles, which then must work harder to stabilize the body and hold it upright. Many spinal injuries and chronic back problems develop because a person's center of gravity moves too far forward, often resulting in too much curvature in the lower back.

A negative attitude exists in our society towards exercising our stomachs, even on the part of people who are well conditioned. It is as if we are repulsed at the idea of exercising our stomachs.

Care of the stomach has other important benefits. Exercising stomach muscles stimulates the digestive organs. They stay in better condition and perform digestion more capably.

BODY MEASUREMENTS

Whether losing weight, building muscle, or for some other reason altering your physical body, one sure way to check your progress is to measure yourself. Measure every six weeks or so to help gauge your progress. The following areas can be evaluated, making sure to measure each area in the same spot each time to ensure accuracy: neck, arms, forearms, chest, waist, hips, thighs, and calves.

SELF-EVALUATION: YOUR BODY IN COMPARISION TO SIX BASIC BODY TYPES

All of us fit into one or more basic body types. Understanding them, in particular the categories you fall into, will be very helpful to any health or exercise program. All body types have advantages and disadvantages as well as fundamental tendencies. Look at the tendencies you have and notice any similarities. Doing so provides understanding of the body in an athletic context.

MEDIAL

The medial body type is considered average. There is nothing unusual about the build, the proportions being excellent. People with medial body types have great all-around capabilities, but because of an inclination to work and play hard, learning to relax would greatly help them. Medials should use their energy on a priority basis and avoid spreading it too thin over a lot of activities. People with this body type can usually learn to do any athletic activity well.

MESO-MEDIAL

The meso-medial body type is a variation of the medial, the only difference being heavier and stronger muscles. The meso-medial is an ideal athlete, possessing all the qualities of the medial, plus added strength. The greatest all-around athletes are of this category. Both medials and meso-medials should pay special attention to flexibility and muscle lengthening, guarding against becoming muscle bound.

MESO-MORPH

The meso-morph is a big, husky type with strong, thick legs, a wide chest, and a narrow waist. Muscles are smooth, though big and strong. The outline of the musculature of this body type is less defined than in the medial or meso-medial. Meso-morphs like body contact and prefer activites in which power and strength are important. They also tend to be somewhat slower and less agile than some other body types. They tend to exercise only when necessary. As they love to eat, meso-morphs are often overweight.

ECTO-MORPH

The ecto-morph is a thinner version of the meso-morph. Ecto-morphic people are usually tall and slim, with long, smooth muscles that are not sharply defined. Because of a lean build, ecto-morphs must take caution against injuries. They benefit by strengthening the muscles as much as possible.

ECTO-MEDIAL

The ecto-medial is the thin, wiry type, usually fast, quick, active and agile. These types do well in high skill activites. Lots of nervous energy inclines them to reach terrific peaks of effort. These people are rarely attracted to hard physical contact, using instead their agility and speed, which is nature's way of protecting them.

ENDO-MORPH

The endo-morph has a rounded-body with narrow shoulders, big buttocks, and hips. The muscles are loose, fatty, and lacking in tone. These people must devote considerable attention to their diets. Physical activity should include speed and hard physical effort that is increased gradually.

Just as important as understanding your body type are the characteristics of various exercises themselves. Many recreational sports and activities provide enjoyment along with physical stimulation necessary for a healthy body. An examination of the more popular forms of exercise can help you decide which activities best suit you.

14

PHYSICAL EXERCISE: ACTIVITIES AND ATHLETICS

"It is not the critic who counts; not the man who points out how the strong man stumbled or where the doer of deeds could have done better. The credit belongs to the man who is actually in the arena; whose face is marred by sweat and dust and blood; who strives valiantly; who errs and comes short again and again; who knows the great enthusiasms, the great devotions, and spends himself in a worthy cause; who at the best, knows the triumph of high achievement; and who, at the worst, if he fails, at least fails while daring greatly so that his place shall never be with those cold and timid souls who knew neither victory nor defeat."

Theodore Roosevelt

Daily activities and athletics run the gamut from walking to triathlons, all of which involve the use of the spine. Warming up the spine is imperative, especially before engaging in contact sports or rigorous training of any kind. Repetition, while not overdoing it and particularly when first starting a program, provides benefits for your body and reduces the chances of injuring yourself. The following activities are discussed in order to explore some of their strengths and weaknesses. They are the more common activities people participate in today.

WALKING

Walking is a fundamental movement. It is a simple exercise to perform and requires only a comfortable pair of shoes and a place to walk. Walking is easy on the joints and the spine. It is an excellent activity, particularly for those who have injured themselves and for the elderly who may experience difficulty in doing other activities.

Walking can provide at least a minimal amount of exercise during the normal course of the day. If you are in very poor shape, walking is a good way to change your condition. Regular walking is a good build-up to more stenuous activites. Try to walk on soft ground whenever possible. This will help cushion the force going into your body. Being outside has other advantages, like fresh air and contact with the world around you. Walking at a brisk pace will provide more conditioning for your body.

If you can, speed walk. Speed walking requires quickening the step. It works your arms, which will speed up your cardio-vascular system. A quicker pace tires you out sooner, but may be just the thing if you really aren't gung ho about exercising. In itself, walking is excellent physical activity.

Walk with good posture. This cannot be emphasized enough. Be conscious of how you walk and give yourself time to make corrective changes. We are creatures of habit, often falling back into old patterns of behavior. This is especially true of walking and other routine activities.

JOGGING - RUNNING

Jogging is defined as running at a slow, leisurely, continuous pace. Many people enjoy jogging regularly as part of their exercise program. It provides excellent cardio-vascular conditioning, particularly over long distances of several miles or more. There is also muscle development of the lower extremities.

Futhermore, people enjoy what is commonly referred to as "runner's high," a euphoric feeling that comes with pushing the body, within reason, over a period of time. The main disadvantage of jogging is that it puts a lot of stress on the spine. You MUST have good posture, no back problems, and know how to jog properly. Otherwise the disadvantages outweigh the benefits. Improper jogging is an example of how ignoring the care of your spine defeats the very purpose of exercising. Jogging should be smooth and flowing, with an element of grace to it.

Running is like jogging, except faster. You get winded much quicker, but it tends to be a more natural pace, especially at about a half or three quarters speed. Here again, posture is a big concern. The right shoes and a proper warm-up beforehand are a must, whether jogging or running.

If you are really serious about jogging and plan to do it regularly, I would suggest consulting with your doctor FIRST about proper posture, shoes, and any special considerations regarding your body and its condition, especially the heart.

Many people have muscular or spinal alignment problems. Jogging just makes them worse. They may start with the best of intentions but wind up being treated for injuries that often could have been prevented in the first place.

The surface you run on also has to be considered. A track has a cushion to it which helps absorb some of the force. Concrete has none. You and your spine, then, absorb all of the force.

SWIMMING

Swimming is possibly the most beneficial physical activity for fitness and restoration of health (Cyriax 104). Swimming offers several advantages not found in other forms of exercise. The reason that swimming is so good is simple: The inherent properties of water and its effect on the body while being submerged in it. In water, our bodies feel as if they are defying gravity, like flying. Most people find the feel of water both pleasurable and soothing. Swimming exercises, and therefore develops, both sides of the body equally.

Water is good for both the skin and the nervous system, providing them with an effective yet non-invasive stimulation. It is becoming more common to treat injuries and disabilities through water related activities (Katz 2-5).

Being in water also eliminates much of the weight-bearing stress of standing in a vertical position. Therefore, there is less stress on the joints during muscle contraction, with the added advantage of having the stress equally distributed throughout the joint, not just in one area. This makes swimming a very theraputic activity.

Every time a runner's foot hits the ground, the shock going into his or her body can be three times the weight of the body. However, a swimmer's body feels as though it weighs less in water, largely due to the force of bouyancy. There is no pounding or jarring against hard surfaces. Moving through the water is a smooth, rhythmic motion.

Swimming comes naturally. It is rare that someone can't be taught to swim. If done properly, swimming develops all three areas of exercise: flexibility, cardio-vascular, and strength. Swimming develops muscles, exercises the heart and lungs, and increases coordination. It can build muscular strength and increase stamina. For getting into shape and staying in shape, swimming is excellent. Forty-five minutes of serious swimming three times a week goes a long way. And besides all the other benefits, swimming has a low incidence of injury.

BICYCLING

Bicycling is a highly beneficial exercise for cardio-vascular conditioning. It has the added advantage of being a source of transportation, which makes it a very practical form of exercise. Riding a bicycle to work or around town can be quite enjoyable. It can provide solitude riding along trails or serve as a social event to share with friends. Many of us rode bicycles as children and would be surprised to find out how easy, fun, and relaxing the sport can be for us as adults.

Riding a bicycle is similar to the way one uses a car's transmission. Progress to the next gear as you steadily build speed. The cadence or pedal speed matters greatly. Keeping it at a high rate benefits your heart, and provides excellent stimulation for the entire cardio-vascular system. Don't lug the gears, the result of a slow pedal speed, especially going uphill. Unnecessary stress is put on the knees.

Bicycling also has disadvantages to consider such as automobile traffic and exhaust. Finding areas with little automobile traffic avoids pollution and reduces the chance of a collision. Posture can be affected by having the shoulders rounded forward for long periods of time. This position isn't good for the spine. Exercises such as bringing your shoulders back and pushing your chest out will help to compensate.

Twisting your spine properly before bicycling is a must. Don't just jump on the bike and take off. First warm up the body, particularly the legs and lower back.

Also, make sure the seat height is adjusted properly. The up and down movement of the legs is critical—the knees should be neither overly bent nor totally straight as you pedal. Ask for consultation at a good bicycle shop to ensure a proper fit, maximizing your conditioning and minimizing your chances of injury.

As in any activity, the type of equipment used is very important. Bicycles are designed for everything from racing to mountain climbing. Be aware of the use you have in mind before purchasing one.

BASEBALL - BASKETBALL RACQUETBALL - TENNIS - SKATING

This group of activites generally provides good exercise. A fair amount of coordination is called for, and development takes place in the areas of strength, cardio-vascular efficiency, and flexibility. A higher rate of injury occurs in these sports, partially due to falling and running into other players and immovable objects.

There is also a problem associated with a constant strain being placed on one part or side of the body. Baseball pitchers, tennis and racquetball players, for example, stress their throwing arm and shoulder. As compensation, massage can be performed on the affected areas before and after the activity.

The body prefers activities that exercise both sides of the body evenly. This prevents overdevelopment on one side with resultant compensation on the other. If you do something that mainly utilizes one side of the body, devise something to do with the unused side to help compensate. Muscles that are specifically used should be warmed up even more. A proper cool down after these or any activity is important because cooling down helps the body unwind and relax. It is the transition between vigorous activity and little or no movement.

SKIING - CROSS COUNTRY AND DOWNHILL

Skiing is a very popular recreational activity that one should not partake in as a weekend warrior. As discussed before, a weekend warrior does very little in the way of exercise and then subjects the body to a tremendous amount of effort that it often can't handle. If you like to ski, get into condition ahead of time. Having flexibility is essential for skiing. Many injuries occur because a skier has not warmed-up his or her body properly. Putting the joints through a full range of motion will warm up the muscles and joints, allowing you to ski with better control and lessen the chances of injury from sudden jolts and falling, common accidents in downhill skiing.

Cross country skiing, because of the slower speeds, does not generate as many injuries as downhill. It is an excellent aerobic activity that develops the cardio-vascular system and works both sides of the body equally.

FOOTBALL - HOCKEY - HARD CONTACT SPORTS

Few activities beat up the body like hard contact sports. Players of these sports are the real warriors of the flesh. No wonder professional football and hockey players have very short career spans. They are a testament to what the human body and spine can be forced to endure and still survive.

I once attended a lecture given by Dr. Fred Cox, a chiropractor and, at that time, the place kicker for the Minnesota Vikings of the National Football League. He showed some before—and after—game X-rays of a defensive lineman's spine. Linemen engage in contact each time the ball is snapped. The forces and concussions they experience in one game would put most of us into our graves.

Here's what Dr. Cox's presentation showed. The before X-ray, a front view, was of a fairly normal looking, straight spine. The after view was completely different. The spine was curved sideways, as if hit with a baseball bat. It was like an instant case of scoliosis. Players can't sustain damage like that on a regular basis for more than a few years. Many injuries never heal properly because they aren't given enough time.

For those who play strenuous recreational activities, proper spinal care is paramount. Regular massage is advisable, as well, to alleviate injuries and sore areas which will help to prevent chronic conditions.

BODYBUILDING - WEIGHTLIFTING

Unquestionably, barbells and the various weight machines available today help build muscle mass. Highly developed and muscular bodies are often the result of dedicated effort over a long period of time. For personal discipline, strength building, or muscle toning, weightlifting is excellent. But the various apparatus must be used properly and only after the body is fully warmed, especially if one is out of shape. Not only the muscles, but also the tendons and ligaments are weak and subject to injury.

The body shouldn't be overpowered with a lot of weight it isn't prepared to handle. Weight lifting is an activity in which technique is vital. You must be careful with weights. Weight belts must be worn around the lower back area to maintain proper spinal curvature. If the lower back straightens out, the loss of curvature reduces its strength factor, and injury becomes imminent.

While muscles look good and strength has its advantages, being muscle bound and otherwise inflexible is a definite liability. This condition is often the result of poor technique.

There are many simple and effective body building exercises you can do at home with and without weights or other equipment. Pushups, chinups, pullups, and similar exercises develop the body and have a low risk factor when done properly.

DANCING - AEROBICS

Dancing in one form or another has been practiced for ages, while aerobics and its variations have only recently emerged on the fitness scene. Many people enjoy dancing for recreation, as an art form, and for fitness. Dancing enhances flexibility and cardio-vascular development.

Aerobic exercises are performed mainly for physical conditioning. Although quite popular, they have a fairly high injury rate. Strenuous aerobics are best performed by those in excellent physical condition. An important factor is the surface on which aerobics are performed. The harder the surface, the more your body must absorb the forces exerted. A proper warm-up is necessary. So is avoiding jerky, torquing movements. Being graceful, smooth and considerate of your body avoids injury while providing the most benefit from the exercise. Low impact aerobics subject the body to less stress, particularly in the legs and lower back. Exercises combining dancing and aerobics are widely popular, fun, and generally safe. Jumping rope is also beneficial and in itself a simple and basic activity.

The key to exercise and physical activity is to put all the joints of the body through a full range of motion. That way, they maintain their capacity to function properly. Remember, too, that the body is inherently smart. If you do the same activity over and over in the same manner, the body learns how to do it using the least effort and minimizing benefits. For this reason, vary your routines and activities. Make sure your program helps maintain flexibility and cardio-vascular development along with developing muscles or losing weight.

What can you do to overcome your obstacles and take better care of yourself? How about starting a buddy system? First decide your own goals and resolutions. Then write them down. Devise a method to keep track of your progress. This information is then shared with somebody who has also developed his or her own set of goals. This is where accountability comes into play. Now you are accountable to somebody else and that person to you.

Regularly discuss your workouts, results, shortfallings, triumphs and tragedies with your buddy. You can motivate each other or provide a kick in the pants if necessary. Both of you have a common interest, bettering yourself physically. Sharing your experiences will make both of you more accountable, plus provide a support system when the inevitable bad days occur.

Try the system with your spouse, somebody you live or work with, or a good friend. It is important that each person set up his or her own ground rules. The reinforcement attained from the buddy system is mutually benefitting.

OVERTRAINING

Overtraining is a major reason why people do not get results or injure themselves when they exercise. Overtraining results from subjecting the body to more activity than it can adequately recover from. The body requires a period of recovery from exercise in which to rebuild itself and become stronger in the process. Physical development does not take place while exercising but during the period of recovery when the body is utilizing the nutrients taken in from the diet.

Part of the problem of overtraining stems from our belief of "no pain no gain." The attitude is that if a little is good, more is better. There is only so much the body can do and then adequately recover from, especially when just starting a workout program. It is far better to coax the body into a physical exercise program than to shock it.

Sometimes our minds get ahead of our bodies. We want to make up for lost time in one day. The initial weeks of an exercise program should acquaint the body with handling physical activity. Even after one has exercised several months or even years, overtraining can still be a factor. If you go more than three workouts without improvement, feel more fatigue, irratibility, or notice an increase in your resting pulse, chances are good you are overtraining.

It is practically a science to know how much exercise to do without overdoing it. You have to listen to your body and be perceptive to the changes it is going through. Remember that internal changes always take place before external ones do.

Don't expect to increase the amount of your exercise workload every time you work out. The body must physiologically adjust to what you are doing to it. During these periods, you cannot lift as much weight or perform as proficiently in your activities.

It is at this critical time of physiological adjustment that many of us throw in the towel and quit. We develop the belief that we are no longer making progress, that our program isn't working. Don't be discouraged. Nothing is wrong. Your body is making internal adjustments which must occur prior to external ones taking place. Because the benefits of exercise are cumulative, every workout is valuable.

A cooling down period is necessary immediately after exercising. Continue moving around at least five minutes to allow your body to recover. Cooling down prevents your blood from pooling in your lower extremities which can cause an abrupt lowering of your blood pressure. When pooling occurs, not enough blood reaches the heart and unconsciousness or even death can result. Runners can finish their workout by walking briskly. Swimmers can tread water for a couple of minutes. The idea is not to finish exercising abruptly, but to taper off, allowing the body to smoothly return to a normal state of functioning.

15

THE FOOD FACTOR

"I've been on a constant diet
for the past two decades.
I've lost a total of 789 pounds.
By all accounts, I should be
hanging from a charm bracelet."

Erma Bombeck

Proper diet and nutrition is an integral part of health. Like everything else related to health, diet is full of myths and misunderstandings. Unfortunately, many Americans have been misled about their diet and the role it plays in their health. There seems to be a new book out on diet every month. As each is found ineffective, it falls by the wayside and we move on to the next. It is obvious that we lack an understanding of proper diet.

The truth is that there is much experts don't know about diet. But as science investigates this subject, there is increasing evidence linking improper diet to the causes of disease.

Many dietary practices have existed for years without anyone being concerned as to whether or not they are correct practices to follow. Likewise, opinions differ regarding nutrition. Some subjects of debate are the role of meat and dairy products in the diet and the validity of such concepts as food combining and fasting.

Let's explore some basic components of diet and some controversial aspects currently being investigated.

Rather than referring to a short term process for the purpose of losing weight, diet actually pertains to food and drink *regularly* consumed. Therefore, all of us diet, that is, we usually eat on a regular basis.

Nutrition is the process of utilizing types and quantities of foods and evaluating and maintaining proper intake of nutrients. Nutrients are compounds needed by the body to maintain life.

Food provides fuel for the body. Our bodies use food like a car uses gas. And just as different cars require different types of gas, we are all not meant to eat the exact same types and quantities of food. Each person has a unique body with varying nutritional requirements. Eating properly requires some thought.

Humans are omnivorous, feeding on both animal and vegetable substances. We, like all animals, are physically adapted to the type of food we eat. In numbers, human teeth are more herbivorous (vegetable feeding) than carnivorous (flesh feeding). Adults have eight incisors, the front teeth; four eye teeth, known as the canines; and twenty molar and premolar teeth. In all we have thirty-two permanent teeth. The incisors are designed for cutting (such food as vegetables), the canine for tearing (such as meat), and molars for grinding (as in grains). The design and numbers of teeth we have are an indicator of the types of foods best suited for human consumption.

Thousands of years ago humans ate simply. Food was basic, unprocessed, and often eaten raw and in season. Though dietary conditions are different in our society today, the makeup of our bodies is essentially the same. When we carelessly expect them to adapt to our changing dietary habits, we suffer the consequences.

For example, storing extra food energy in the body as fat was a biological survival mechanism. Today, because we eat so regularly, overeating and storing excessive amounts of food energy (fat) is unnecessary and leads to being overweight. Because of improved production and marketing methods, refrigeration, transportation, processing, and chemicals, we have more dietary choices today, regardless of the time of the year. But with these increased choices come unhealthful aspects requiring discretion about what we eat and drink.

THE COMMERCIAL FACTOR

Advertising in our society has programmed us to believe that if food looks good, we should eat it. Food is portrayed as entertainment. The truth is that food is big business. The intention is to create profits, not to serve our health.

As consumers, we must change our attitudes and beliefs about food in order for business to respond. When we give no thought beyond our eyes and taste buds to what we eat, we create health problems for ourselves.

Greater attention is now being focused on the contents of food products. Nutritional labeling is beginning to provide such information. Despite their limitations and abuse of terms (such as "natural"), food product labels are a good place to begin educating yourself about what you are eating.

Some food producers and suppliers supply pamphlets on nutrition and food preparation. Be careful. This information is advertising in disguise. What is *not* stated may be detrimental to your particular condition. For example, although avocados and peanuts are nutrituous, they are also high in fat.

Organizations such as the American Heart Association provide excellent dietary guidelines that can be easily incorporated into one's buying and eating habits. Their recommendations are increasingly found in restaurants.

Nutrition starts at the point of purchase. Here, prudent choices, coupled with good cooking and eating habits, provide the foundation for a healthy diet.

CALORIES

Often despised, calories are simply the measurement of energy in food. Remember, *excess* food energy is stored as fat. This is why the amount of calories one consumes on a daily basis is a factor in our diets.

Knowing some of the commonly used terms associated with calories can guide your choices about what foods you eat. For example, "nutrient density" refers to the amount of nutrients contained in food relative to the number of calories. Nutrient dense foods provide large amounts of nutrients for the calories they contain.

Likewise, "empty" calories applies to low quality foods, commonly known as junk food, that contain a lot of calories but few nutrients. Not getting enough calories from your diet can also be a problem, as you are not getting enough of the nutrients you need on a daily basis.

TOXICITY

Throughout history, prosperous civilizations like ancient Rome and others have had to face the problem of food toxicity. Royalty who ate rich foods in great quantity developed certain diseases, while the peasants, eating a simple diet, did not.

Nowadays, when our processed and devitalized western foods are introduced to different parts of the world, our diet related diseases often follow. Since the body can process and eliminate only so much food and waste on a daily basis, it becomes overburdened by these inferior products. Unfortunately in our country, toxicity is becoming more common in children. Because of parental habits, the influence of advertising, and freedom to purchase and consume what they please, children develop patterns that lead to problems in adulthood.

When an excessive amount of sugar, salt, fat, cholesterol, and man-made chemicals fill our tissues and blood stream, our bodies show it. We become overweight and toxic. Instead of nourishing health, we nourish disease.

How many overweight animals are there on earth? Have you ever heard of a fat eagle or an obese tiger? There are no overweight animals in the wild. The only animals with a weight problem are those that live with people. What does that say about us?

Something must be wrong. The problem is not with our bodies. It's with the way we treat them. Fully one fourth of all adults (about 40 million) in the United States are obese—twenty per cent above ideal weight (Nieman 17). Many of these people will eventually develop serious health problems. Our habits, lack of education about our bodies and the principles of diet, and our apathy are the culprits.

NUTRIENTS

The nutrients required by the body fall into six categories: water, carbohydrates, protein, fat, vitamins, and minerals.

One neglected aspect of health maintenance is water. Our bodies are composed of approximately 60% water. After air, water is the best purifier of the body.

We take water for granted. But it's time we start taking it seriously. We need water for survival. How much of it today is tainted? Since our planet is a closed system, it's only a matter of time until all of our water is polluted. This unfortunate situation prompts the addition of even more chemicals into the water to offset the effects of pollutants.

Drinking several glasses of good *quality* water (as free as possible from chemicals and contaminants) daily is essential to good health. With all the various commercial drinks available today, few of us drink enough water.

Water is especially beneficial to the body in the morning, before you eat or drink anything else. Throughout the night the kidneys filter blood, removing impurities. Drinking water in the morning flushes the kidneys out. In this manner, you're assisting your body's natural cleansing process.

Be careful not to consume too much water or other liquids while eating. When digestive juices become diluted, the digestive process is impeded.

The body also receives water from high water content food, of which fruits and vegetables are the two best sources. The merits of various foods is often argued, but no one questions the value and necessity of eating fruits and vegetables. They are the most natural foods on earth.

A good source of nourishment, fiber, and energy, fruits and vegetables are easily digestable and help clean the body. The more we eat, the better.

Like water, fruit goes through the system quickly as a natural cleanser and energizer. After resting and repairing itself all night, the body needs what fruit has to offer. Fruit gets the digestive system moving again and prepares it to receive more food.

Unfortunately, fruits and vegetables are often treated as a side order or trimming in our diet, an appetizer before serious eating begins. The truth is that fruits and vegetables *are* serious eating.

Complex carbohydrates supply good nutrition, fiber, and energy for the body without adding excess weight. When in their natural state or as unprocessed as possible, their long chains of molecules provide a steady supply of energy for the body and an even metabolism. Whole grains such as wheat, bran, oats, rice, and potatoes are among the main staples of the world and can be served in an endless variety of ways.

Simple carbohydrates such as sugar burn quickly in the body. They rob the body of nutrients and take the metabolism on a roller coaster ride. Bleaching makes food lighter, fancier, and more eye appealing, thus more profitable for the manufacturer. Refined foods separate out parts of the grains they come from and in the process, often remove necessary nutrients and fiber. The main reason for eating—nutritive value—is lost with refined foods.

Enriching foods is an attempt to restore nutrients lost in processing. Advertisers will try to convince you that adding enrichments results in a better product. But once the integrity of wholesome food is destroyed in processing, man-made nutrients can rarely restore it. That is why so many nutritionally conscious people prefer whole, unprocessed foods.

Protein comes from the Greek word meaning "of prime importance" and, next to water, is the most abundant substance in the body. Proteins are the building blocks or structural material in cells. Proteins also act as enzymes that regulate metabolic reaction and, in certain instances, are used to supply energy.

The role of protein in the American diet is a hotly debated subject. The debate centers on how much protein to eat and from what sources.

Eating meat every day has long been a tradition in our society. Supplemented with various dairy products, meat has been a main source of protein. Some people believe that meat eaters are healthier, that meat protein is the ultimate food. For many, a meal isn't a meal without meat.

A daily intake of meat, however, is not necessary for healthy sustenance. Meat is a complete protein which contains valuable amino acids. Only a small amount of it is required to fill most of our protein needs. A highly concentrated food, meat takes a long time and a lot of energy to digest. It often contains man-made growth hormones, additives for tenderness and color, preservatives, and other non-food chemicals. With all of this comes its own high fat and cholesterol content.

A main concern about protein is getting too much in the diet, especially when it comes from eating a lot of red meat. Though we cannot store protein and must have it on a regualr basis, too much protein causes excess work for the kidneys to eliminate what isn't needed.

According to the RDA (Recommended Daily Allowance), a person needs eight tenths of a gram of protein per kilogram of body weight. For example, a person who weighs 150 pounds (68 kilograms, arrived at by dividing pounds by 2.2) requires 54 grams of protein per day. An ounce of red meat contains seven grams of protein. A cup of skim milk provides eight grams. How much protein does *your* body need daily? How much are you consuming now?

The body can assimilate only about thirty grams of protein effectively at a time. Eating small amounts of protein throughout the day is better than consuming large amounts all at once.

As a source of protein and an alternative to red meat, fish and seafood are becoming more popular. Overall, they have less fat and cholesterol, and the body digests them easier. Fish is available in great variety and can be cooked very imaginatively. Fish, however, frequently live in increasingly polluted waters. We hear of fish contaminated with mercury, lead, and other unhealthful chemicals. Be selective when purchasing fish, the same as you would with red meat. Compare varieties and quality found at specialty and health food stores with those of conventional markets.

The second major source of protein in our western diet is dairy foods, which include milk, cheese, yogurt, and eggs. These foods have traditionally been major staples providing protein, vitamins, and minerals.

Many of us have been taught that dairy products are good for us, the more the better. The over consumption of dairy products, however, can cause fat and cholesterol to build up in the bloodstream and body tissues resulting in an increase in susceptibility to heart disease.

Since both meat and dairy products have a limit to their value in the diet, deriving the nutritional value they provide from other food sources is the key to good health. Combinations such as brown rice and legumes (beans, peas, lentils) are such protein sources.

Similiar in composition to carbohydrates, fats are a concentrated source of energy. They yield nine calories per gram and play an important role in our diet. Insulation and temperature regulation for the body are among the functions of fat. Fat acts as an energy source (fats *are* stored energy) and a source of transportation for fat soluable vitamins. Fat intake should be kept at a moderate level, about 30% or less of your total caloric intake.

Cholesterol is a form of fat found only in foods of animal origin. Cholesterol is a part of bile, which is secreted by the liver and is necessary in the digestion of fats. Certain hormones are composed, in part, of cholesterol. Cholesterol plays a role in the structure of brain and nerve cells.

Since cholesterol can be manufactured by the body, it is not considered an essential nutrient. Many of the foods we eat today, however, contain cholesterol.

The problem is not so much that cholesterol is in food, but what happens when too much of it gets into your blood. When it does, it narrows the arteries, setting the stage for atherosclerosis—hardening of the arteries.

Vitamins and minerals are part of a good diet. Both benefit the body in specific ways. Vitamins are potent, organic, noncaloric compounds. Their functions include promoting growth and reproduction. Minerals function as constituents of both hard and soft tissues and assist in the regulation of body functions.

Vitamins and minerals are optimally obtained by eating raw, live, and unprocessed foods in their most natural state. Don't eat junk food and then try to compensate with large doses of vitamins. Your body is then burdened with the task of removing excessive toxins, the result of nutritionally deficient by-products in junk food.

Like all nutrients, vitamins and minerals have to be first digested before being assimilated. You may have to experiment with different types to find those that are compatible to your system. Vitamins, however, should be considered a supplement to the diet, not the sole source of your nutrition. They do not contain fiber, water, and other nutrients necessary for proper bodily function.

Reasonable amounts of vitamin and mineral supplements are like a form of insurance, compensating for anything your regular diet is lacking. Take vitamins with meals for proper absorption of nutrients.

FIBER

Fiber includes the indigestible components in food that help expedite the digestive process. Whole grains, fruits, and vegetables are among the major contributors of fiber to the diet. Not having enough fiber can lead to digestive disorders caused by matter staying in the digestive system too long. Likewise, the risk of exposure of the digestive tract walls to cancer-causing agents in food is increased. Having too much fiber can limit the absorption of certain nutrients.

HERBS

Herbs include any plant or plant part valued for medicinal or savory qualities. They are used primarily for food seasoning and drinks, medical treatment, and nutritional value. Mustard is a commonly used herb. So are many of the spices found in people's kitchens used as seasoning. Historically, the medicinal uses of herbs have been most important.

Throughout much of history, man possessed limited resources with which to combat injuries and ailments. Plant remedies have been the most universal and enduring forms of health care treatment. Many have been found to have positive effects on the body when consumed in small amounts.

In herbs, nutrients are stored within the plant's cellular structure. These nutrients are easily metabolized by the gastric juices, enzymes, and hormones of your body. Most herbs have to be consumed regularly to obtain their beneficial effects. Store them in airtight containers away from heat, light, and dampness. Proper storage prevents deterioration of the active ingredients. Take care: Some herbs can be potent. Overdoses can create adverse side effects.

16

OUR EATING HABITS

"Eat to live, and not live to eat.
Many dishes, many diseases.
To lengthen thy life, lessen thy meals.
Who is strong?
He who can conquer his bad habits."

Benjamin Franklin

Our health is affected by not only what, but how, we eat. Eating habits start early in life. Take a look at what your eating habits are and how they began. Who can deny the difficulty faced by someone who grew up on a bad diet? Habits, formed through years of ingrained behavior, do not vanish overnight. They take time to change. Start by reducing and replacing the wrong foods with the right ones. You can succeed if you persist.

A well balanced diet has variety, a critical factor too often overlooked. Sometimes we find ourselves eating the same few foods day after day. To eat an apple a day and call that eating fruit is not enough. Eating a variety of foods allows you to take advantage of each food's unique nutritional qualities.

No dietary change becomes permanent unless you integrate it into your lifestyle. It's a fact. Constant changing of diets, trying this and that, goes on year after year. Your stomach and budget get abused in the process. Start looking at your lifestyle and understand the basic axioms of good diet. Then do the best you can. That way, you are taking control.

Your tongue quickly tells you whether or not you like something. It becomes conditioned to the types of food you eat. If you eat a lot of salty or sugary food, your tongue and body will react if you suddenly quit. Everything will taste bland because the food is not as tasty as before. If you gradually cut down on the use of salt and sugar, however, the tastebuds become reconditioned and can begin to distinguish the different, natural tastes of the foods you eat. Be consistent. Give yourself credit every step of the way. Realize that many habits are unconscious. We must understand why we have them and then gradually change our behavior.

We love to add flavoring to the food we eat. Pancakes, for example, are often flavored with butter and syrup. Instead of saying you can't use the butter or syrup, go easy on them. Use natural, unsalted butter and real maple syrup instead of the artificial kind.

Another habit is drowning salad in dressing. Since many commercial salad dressings are high in fat and loaded with chemicals, go easy on them. Try a salad sprinkled with an unsalted herbal seasoning or lemon juice. Experiment. Try making your own or consider the many low calorie dressings now available. Read through some natural food cookbooks. Rather than feeling bad about denying yourself something, compliment yourself for using self-control and self-discipline. Feel good about yourself for daring to break undesirable patterns. Your new behavior will become habit forming. Remember, you don't have to give up your favorite goodies entirely. Simply use less or find better quality substitutes. You'll enjoy them all the more.

Eating your food slowly and chewing it well is also an important dietary habit. Some of us eat like vacuum cleaners, which causes the food to pile up in the stomach and sit there. When you eat too fast, your body doesn't get the chance to tell you to stop eating until you have already eaten too much.

Proper digestion of food, including liquids, begins in the mouth. Salivary glands in the mouth aid digestion by moistening food particles, binding them together, beginning the digestion of carbohydrates, and dissolving food so it can be tasted. By eating too fast, digestion does not begin until the food is in your stomach. You can save yourself digestive problems and better enjoy eating when you eat slowly and chew your food thoroughly.

Changing cooking habits can also benefit your diet. Overcooking foods causes a loss of nutrients. Instead of boiling vegetables, lightly steam them. Save the water for later use as soup stock.

There is a big difference between cooking whole grains and bleached products. White rice is processed to cook fast and puff up at the expense of nutrients. Natural brown rice is heavier. You should rinse all grains, lentils, rice, and the like before cooking to remove dirt and residue.

Nut butters in their natural state separate since there are no chemical stabilizers added. Stir them when you first open the jar and store them in the refrigerator. Fruits and vegetables should be washed well with a grease cutting soap to remove pesticides and wax.

BREAKING OLD HABITS

Most of us have some favorite fruits and vegetables. They're a good place to start to improve your diet. Realize that you may now like foods you didn't in the past. How many times have you not eaten something because you didn't like it the first time you tried it? How long ago was that? Try again and find out if it tastes better to you now.

How can you like good, natural food if your whole life has been a diet of processed, salted, and sugared food? People say, "I can't stomach the taste of that." Well, they can't. Their taste buds are conditioned to what they are used to eating. Anything else won't taste as flavorful.

Conversely, someone who eats a lot of fresh foods can't tolerate eating canned and processed food. A slow but sure move away from processed foods makes the most difference over the long term. Why eat well one week and then poorly the next?

Look to the psychological aspects of diet for an explanation. Remember when you were a child? When something bad happened, were you comforted with cookies or candy? Sweets and junk food are often used as bribes or reward mechanisms with children to control or otherwise change their behavior. This continues throughout life. We reach for certain types of food when we feel unloved, under stress, or depressed.

I find it quite ironic to see what's being sold in supermarkets today. Most of the larger chains have a small aisle labeled "Health/Nutrition." Well, if that's what's on that aisle, what is on the other aisles? What is the rest of the food they are selling supposed to be?

As long as the junk food stays on the grocery store shelf, you're safe. When it's put into your shopping cart, you're in trouble. Once you bring it home, you lose. Who buys food with the intention of not eating it? What is the first thing we eat when we come home from shopping? The so-called goodies, naturally.

To avoid temptation, shop when you're not hungry. Think about what you really need. Make yourself at home in the produce aisle, among the fresh fruits and vegetables. Utilize a variety of grains, lentils, and beans, as well as lean meat, fish and fowl. Plan your meals from a nutritional point of view. Don't let your eyes, taste buds and susceptibility to advertising lead you astray.

Eat conscientiously. Then you can afford not to be as picky when choices are limited, as in restaurants. You can eat the foods you like but no longer eat at home. It's a process of replacing negative eating habits with sound nutritional ones.

When you are eating properly on a day-to-day basis, you can afford to treat yourself once in awhile. The trick is not to make yourself wrong when you do. You can overlook the occasional treat or indulgence without getting down on yourself, eliminating unnecessary guilt. We all fall short of the mark occasionally. Understanding this fact of life is also part of the truth about health. When you can do that, you're really in charge of your health and your life.

WEIGHT CONTROL

Millions of dollars are made from overweight people who try every conceivable way possible to shed a few pounds. The gimmicks used on us by advertisers work on our egos and vanity through peer pressure.

Being overweight can result from many factors. One is too many calories, often the result of a diet high in fats and junk food. The average diet today contains many foods that are primarily empty calories and low in nutrient density.

Lack of adequate physical activity is another reason why people are overweight. The energy from food must be used; otherwise it is stored as fat. Ignorance of proper dietary habits or blatant disregard for the natural laws that govern us and the world we live in can be a particular downfall.

Physical activity is a critical factor in weight control. Simple common sense tells you that the more a person weighs, the harder his or her body works. Too much weight makes it difficult to be active. One tires very easily, a condition that reinforces inactivity. It's a self-defeating cycle.

For snacks, enjoy the natural goodness of fruits and vegetables. If you always have them available at home and at work, you'll be less tempted to snack on junk food. Use a smaller dinner plate, thereby making portions appear larger.

Eat desserts sparingly, a way to limit problem foods without completely depriving yourself. Many of your favorite desserts can be made without sugar and other low nutrient, high calorie ingredients. Seek out cookbooks concerned with the *quality* as well as the taste of food.

Make a list of a half dozen of your highest calorie weaknesses. Replace them with healthier items that you like. Realize that you're in control.

Weigh yourself every week instead of every day. This practice eliminates normal daily fluctuations that may frustrate you. Regardless of how much weight you want to lose, the facts are still the same. Losing a pound of fat means burning 3500 calories more than you consume—another reason why physical activity is an important factor in weight control.

Three to four weekly workouts, a half hour or more in length, is quite optimal for maintaining fitness or losing weight. Aerobic exercises like swimming, bicycling, walking, or running, as well as structured exercise classes, burn calories most efficiently. You may become less sensitive to stress as a result of exercising regularly. Reducing stress may help cut down on overeating. The discipline of pushing yourself away from the table after you know you've had enough is an excellent starting point.

Emotional well-being is important to the overall health of any individual. Emotional problems often manifest themselves in diet and eating habits. Food consumption compensates for emotional problems by acting as a reward or compensation mechanism. Here again is a case of treating symptoms rather than causes. Professional assistance in dealing with the emotional aspect of weight control can help one get to the source of a problem and correct it.

Being overweight is a serious cause of stress on the spine. The spine is burdened by excess fat that tends to collect around the abdomen, disrupting the normal distribution of weight. The extra weight adds tremendous strain to your spinal column and lower back, in particular. If the overweight condition continues for a long time, chronic problems can develop.

Be confident that the permanent dietary changes you are making are beneficial to your health over the long term. Give yourself credit for your efforts of self-improvement. Have faith that you are doing the right thing. You are!

The speed in which one loses weight also has to be taken into account. Naturally, we would like to lose our excess weight all at once. Many even try to lose weight by literally starving themselves. The body functions best when weight loss is no more than one to two pounds per week. This tends to be a contradiction to people. Intellectually, we want to lose more than is realistic. Undoubtably it took time to put the extra weight on. During that process, the body had to make periodic internal adjustments. The same is true with losing weight. The body must adjust internally to the changes being made (fewer calories, more exercise) before you see external improvements.

Look at it this way. Let's say you could lose two pounds a week, week in week out. If that isn't fast enough for you consider that in three months, you will have lost about twenty-five pounds. That increases to fifty pounds in six months. If you kept it up for a year, it would be a whopping one hundred pounds. Additionally, your body easily adjusts to this slow and steady change, which reduces your chances of putting the weight back on.

INTERNAL MAINTENANCE

Resting the body's digestive organs and maintaining a level of internal cleanliness are two other important factors in maintaining health. We eat or digest food virtually every hour of the day. Some of us cannot sleep without a midnight snack. Digesting food is serious work for your body, as it must expend a lot of energy in the process. As with anything else, when the internal organs are periodically rested, they function better and last longer.

Do you leave your car running all the time? That is precisely what happens to your body when you eat from morning until night. Even though you rest nightly, the digestive system is still working. The digestive organs rest only after you haven't eaten food for several hours. When there is no food left to digest, the body then directs more of its attention towards internal cleansing.

While you sleep at night, your body does its cleansing, repairing, and healing. That is why you have bad breath and body odor in the morning and need to eliminate waste. Your body has been ridding itself of potential disease-causing waste products.

Have you ever seen the inside of an automobile engine when the oil had never been changed? There is an accumulation of sludge and dirt, making it hard for the moving parts to perform well. A similiar occurrence can take place inside the body. Without proper diet and exercise habits, excess fats, cholesterol, and poisons can overwhelm the body's capacity to eliminate them.

What we eat is not the only issue here. When drugs, smoking, and environmental pollution are taken into account, it is inevitable that toxins find their way into the body. The question becomes how to eliminate them on a regular basis and avoid becoming overly toxic.

The body has a limited capacity to remove toxins from its system. Our modern way of eating rich and chemically saturated foods frequently exceeds that capacity.

What happens to your system when it contains too many toxins? The body can only take so much before it gets sick. What matters is getting rid of the toxins before your body becomes overwhelmed by them. In part, your body gets sick in order to eliminate excessive toxins and keep you well.

When an animal becomes sick, it stops eating and concentrates its energy cleansing its system. Whatever is causing the discomfort is removed. Human beings have the same natural inclinations. How many times have you been sick and not wanted to eat? What do you think your body was trying to tell you? It was saying, "Give me a break!"

When the body is trying to clean itself, allow it to do so. Plenty of rest and drinking of fluids, particularly water and fresh fruit juices, will help the body perform its natural healing processes.

17

CHALLENGES TO HEALTH

"Everything in excess is opposed by nature."

Hippocrates

Life today contains many challenges to our health. They include the vices and habits that predominate in society and which are intensified by the condition of the environment and the way we take care of ourselves. Let's explore four main challenges to health: genetic, environmental, iatrogenic, and lifestyle.

GENETIC

Heredity is the transmission of genetic information from parents to offspring. Genetic information, or genes, are passed in the form of DNA molecules contained in the nuclei of sperm and egg cells, providing chemical instructions for human development.

Genes cause children to resemble as well as to differ from their parents, becoming unique individuals with characteristics of their own. Genetics accounts for and includes the similarities and differences between parents and their offspring and the mechanisms responsible for them.

Contained within each of our bodies are hereditary tendencies or predispositions that affect our health and longevity. Some children are born with disabilities or diseases, or will develop various health problems later in life due to genetics. Each situation presents its own challenge.

Often a family predisposition toward a particular disease or group of diseases may exist. While this is no guarantee that one will have the affliction, the chances of contracting it are greater. This is why doctors take individual and family histories. If your family has a history of such things as heart trouble or cancer, it may necessitate being checked for them on a regular basis.

While some people's health can legitimately be impaired because of hereditary factors, that condition is no excuse to perpetuate negative attitudes and bad habits. Our bodies have a great capacity to adapt and compensate for shortcomings.

ENVIRONMENTAL

Environment includes the chemical, physical, and biological factors that act to influence every individual's life. Our environment is what we depend on for our survival as individuals and as a species. Unfortunately, the environment today is not conducive to good health.

Look at the condition of our planet. In the name of so-called development and progress we are destroying the environment. Toxic waste dumps and air and water pollution upset the earth's ecology. Increasing numbers of industrial mishaps contribute to the problem. Major chemical and nuclear disasters destroy life and permanently scar the earth. The same is true of the terrorist attacks and war which have become commonplace on our planet.

Other environmental hazards are subtle and not easily detected or measured. It is hard to gauge their effect on the body or the body's ability to adapt to them. Such a problem today is the prevalence of stress in our lives.

Stress severely challenges our health; handling it is vital to survival. How you manage stress is more important than how much you have. That is why some people can cope with high pressure jobs for years, while others have difficulty buying groceries.

The major by-product of stress is tension. Tension prohibits muscular relaxation. Part of the normal functioning of our muscles is to stay relaxed when not in use. Muscles that cannot relax are always in a state of contraction and stay tight. Over a period of time they begin to shorten, losing their ability to relax and release tension.

Part of our problem with handling stress is due to our natural defense mechanism, the "fight or flight syndrome." Centuries ago, when confronted with a stressful situation, we had two choices: to fight or to flee. Thus the body has a built-in mechanism governing its priority of action when placed under stress. Today, however, that stress-releasing process is often stifled in our civilized society. Rather than fighting or fleeing, we must contain ourselves and stew in our anger and frustration. Thus, the pressures of daily life build up rather than decrease right at the time they occur.

Everyone deals with stress in an individual way. Some methods, such as physical exercise and relaxation techniques, are effective in relieving stress. Others—excessive smoking, drugs, and alcohol—become avoidances which in being used to mask the problem only contribute to it.

Stress comes in two forms: short-term and long-term. Short-term stress deals with basic survival, such as waiting in line, fighting traffic, or losing your wallet.

Long term stress involves issues of longer duration such as being in debt, losing your job, or dissolving a close relationship.

Managing stress means relaxing under pressure. You must be able to vent your negative energies and frustrations that continually build up. Physical exercise or a good massage, a hot shower, or soothing bath are excellent ways to relax. Breathing exercises and meditation are immensely valuable. When at your wit's end, screaming your heart out into your pillow will allow you to blow your stack—safely.

Continually coping with stress demands a reliable process of emotional expression. Talking to oneself, a friend, or a professional can serve this purpose and will help to put the mind and body at ease. When bottled up emotionally, we are bottled up physically. A habit of regular physical exercise may help you break this impasse and relieve your emotional stress.

IATROGENIC

The word iatrogenic comes from the Greek word *iatro,* meaning "doctor," and *genic* which means "produced." Iatrogenic diseases are side effects resulting from the application of drugs prescribed by a doctor.

Every drug—even the mildest forms such as aspirin—has side effects. Sometimes, prescribing medicine becomes a guessing game of whether the side effect from a drug is better or worse than the patient's original symptoms.

Many people fail to inform their doctors fully about the kinds and amount of medication they are taking. Drugs react differently when taken in combination with others. Depending on body chemistry, they also have various effects on a person's body.

A drug may be tested and meet certain requirements, but the true test is when it is dispensed to the masses. It often takes years before the real side effects show up. This is playing chemical warfare with our own bodies.

Our "pill for every problem" consciousness is the real culprit. We want a fix for everything, refusing to accept even the slightest discomfort. Advertising merely reinforces this habit by pounding into our heads how relief is only a swallow away. For the sake of profit, our health is further endangered by chemicals that can do us more harm than the problem we have in the first place.

As drugs become more powerful, they have a greater ability to change the chemical and physiological make-up of the human body. So we trade off seemingly miraculous improvements on one hand for potentially disasterous consequences on the other.

Nosocomial disease is related to iatrogenic since it refers to problems associated with hospital care. Hospitals are breeding grounds for infections, as germs are transmitted from one patient to another by the hospital staff. Contaminated rooms and instruments also play a major role in the spread of disease, as do errors in medication and anaesthesia. Although many patients are being kept alive longer, their delicate conditions and the prevalence of surgical wounds make them more susceptible to infections (Cherry 96 and Gilbert 34).

Remember the swine flu? Health authorities decided that only a vaccine could save us. A lot of us took it. Some people got sick, some died. The point is that the vaccine didn't work. It was not the solution to the cause, but a random shot in the dark. Everything has been tampered with, even the most basic experiences of human life, such as giving birth.

The process of birth is a challenge to life itself. Birth is often a semi-surgical procedure. Twenty per cent of all births in America today are Caesarian section: one reason being obstetricians fear the threat of lawsuits resulting from natural birth complications (Clark 31).

Mothers are often drugged during labor to ease their pain and make the process easier. Often, forceps replace the mother's active assistance in delivering the baby. This plier-like instrument attaches behind the baby's ears and literally pulls the baby out of the mother's body. Since the neck and spinal cord of a newborn are so fragile, the use of forceps can be dangerous.

Who can deny that life will have its moments of discomfort? Trying to mask over every problem with some newfangled drug is not the answer. If it were, we would have found a cure for everything by now and life would all be a bed of roses. Maybe it's time we do a little honest examination of our own habits.

LIFESTYLE

Discussing our personal habits can get touchy. We tend to be defensive about what we do. It's obvious we are not perfect by the way we treat ourselves, one another, and the world around us. What we must realize, however, is that our imperfections and habits greatly influence our health. You don't have to be perfect to be healthy.

Not having to be perfect to be healthy means reaching beyond our imperfections. Society programs us to think and believe that certain habits are acceptable while others are not. This programming has no effect on the body, however. Your body deals strictly with what you do to and with it. It makes no difference that some chemicals we ingest are legal while others are not. The principle is still the same. The choice is up to us.

AGEING: DESTINY OR DECISION?

Our attitudes about ageing are reflected by our beliefs. They shape our experiences as we get older. Our mental conceptions are thus lived out physically. For this reason, ageing must be understood from both its mental and physical aspects.

What are your thoughts on ageing? An inevitable occurrence that can't be helped? But is that the truth? How did you arrive at such an opinion?

The formation of your beliefs started when you were young. You probably saw Grandma and Grandpa or other elderly people, gray haired, frail, and not in full control of their faculties. As you grew up, did you assume the same would happen to you?

Did you ever wonder why or how ageing happens as it does? Many believe that by the time they're thirty or forty years of age, they are over the hill, their bodies shot. It's time we compare our old conceptions with some fresh, new data.

Though many of us get old long before our time, the 1984 Summer Olympic Games provided a superb example of life's physical potential. Many participants were at or near their maximum capabilities while still in their teens or early twenties. Each event placed different demands on the athlete. One example is the 26 mile, 385 yard marathon race.

The marathon requires a combination of both speed and endurance. Can you imagine running that distance without a stop? Forget the 26 miles. Could you run the 385 yards? The training for such an event is grueling, to say the least. A lot can happen during the time it takes to run such a distance. Understandably, many participants completely fatigue and drop out of the race.

The start of the 1984 Olympic marathon focused attention on the favored runners. But someone else was to win on that hot, smoggy day in Los Angeles: Carlos Lopes of Portugal. He was thirty-seven. Evidently, he didn't know he was too old to be a winner.

By thirty-seven, how many people think that the old bones just aren't what they used to be? On his victory, Carlos remarked, "It was my youthfulness and endurance." Youthfulness at thirty-seven? Yes. It was his belief about his age that counted. His actions and results naturally followed. He is not the only example.

Every year the sport of bicycling stages an event called The Race Across America. It starts in Huntington Beach, California, at the edge of the Pacific Ocean. Many enter and ride along for the first 100 miles, a considerable distance. The race continues on, however, to Atlantic City, New Jersey, ending at the Atlantic Ocean.

Those who have experienced driving a car that distance know how exhausting the task can be. How about doing that on a bicycle? Pedaling more than 3,000 miles is pretty serious physical activity. Only those in excellent shape could attempt such a feat. How old could someone like that be? Only the young need apply, right? The winner in 1986, Pete Penseyres, set a new record, riding his bicycle across America in 8 days, 9 hours and 47 minutes. He was forty-three. His victory was no fluke, as he had also won the race in 1984.

Our bodies age as fast as we let them. In reality these people are the fit ones. The rest of us have fallen far, far behind. Our effort to retain youthfulness and health calls for more commitment as we grow older. If you say all that effort isn't for you, fine. But understand, you CAN do something about ageing.

Let me introduce a personal anecdote here. My Aunt Theresa was the first person I met who was old in years but young in mind and body. When I was nine, my parents went away for a few days and Aunt Theresa came to stay with us. She was past seventy. My parents made it clear that we would be on our best behavior, as Aunt Theresa couldn't be expected to handle things as well as my mother, thirty years her junior.

It was immediately apparent to me that my aunt was as capable as my mother. She was neither slow nor hard of hearing; all her faculties were in good working order. There was good reason for this. Aunt Theresa was a practicioner of sound, healthy habits.

We started every morning with a glass of purified water, then a fresh fruit salad. Aunt Theresa prepared almost everything from scratch. In fact, she was quite upset at my sister's suggestion that a can of ravioli would be fine for lunch.

At that time I questioned this drastic change in our eating habits. Why was Aunt Theresa making everything herself and serving so much raw food? We ate fine before she came along, I thought. Aunt Theresa even brought along her own bottled water, claiming the chemicals in ordinary tap water were unhealthful. I wondered if my parents really knew this person they had left to care for their children.

My aunt held strong convictions about health. She explained to me how they came about. About thirty years prior, Aunt Theresa had attended a seminar given by Dr. Paul Bragg, a life extension specialist. Dr. Bragg taught the importance of developing a quality relationship between the mind, body, and environment. This relationship was based on maintaining a proper diet of natural, unprocessed foods, quality drinking water, and a program of regular physical exercise. It was Dr. Bragg's all encompassing philosophy that had captivated my aunt.

Dr. Bragg believed the human body functioned due to a built-in vital force with which we must cooperate in order to stay healthy. Dr. Bragg was living proof of his own principles, which demonstrated how mankind can have greater control over health and ageing. He believed that life was meant to be like a candle, burning brightly from start to finish, sputtering once or twice, then quickly going out.

Because of the effect of Dr. Bragg's teachings, my Aunt Theresa questioned the belief that we must slow down as we age, get sick, and die a slow death. I then realized an important truth about health.

Although staying healthy takes effort, especially as one gets older, the rewards are vast. You may not want to put that much effort into maintaining your health, but don't say it can't be done. Instead, say that you choose not to. We all die eventually, but some of us use that fact as a license not to care about our health.

Health is best understood with awareness of the big picture, what all the pieces are and how they fit together. We have covered a lot of ground, yet have just scratched the surface. While there is so much we still have to learn, there is much we already know and should utilize for the benefit of all. It's imperative we quit applying short term solutions to long range problems.

18

YOUR SPINE, YOUR MIND, OUR TIMES

Health is:
Education to develop
Awareness,
Love of self and others,
Truth, and the state of
Happiness

As a child, I watched my father suffer, his daily existence a struggle against a disease that never let up, would never relent or go away. His condition and its effect on my life was all encompassing.

Growing up, my interest intensified for the truth about health. I found out quickly that health care is a business. The biggest reason why there is so much furor over our health today, in a word, is money. Health is a big issue and also a lot of ground to cover. My book has touched upon some key areas. My greatest wish is that you, too, will be able to go out and cover some ground. Understanding enough facts about the body (yours in particular) and how it works is the basis for properly taking care of yourself. Ultimately, three crucial factors are self-responsibility, practical knowledge, and common sense.

Our world faces difficult challenges. Most of us would like to do something about them. The question is, what? How can we as individuals measurably affect the world around us? And where does one begin? The subject of health, especially our own, is an excellent starting point. Health provides the ability we have to experience life itself. It determines both our individual condition and that of the planet as a whole. Health is so valuable that no amount of money could ever buy it.

Health is much simpler to comprehend when reduced to its basic components. The maintenance of the master control center, the spine (brain, spinal cord, and spinal column) profoundly affects a person's overall condition. We must take personal action with an attitude of accountability.

We are fortunate that taking care of the spine—a delicate, complex, and irreplaceable organ—is so simple. Care of the spine does not require a great expense of energy, time, or money.

People with the gumption to have some interest in their own health should be applauded. They are taking steps to ensure a sound future for themselves, not just hoping it will happen.

SUFFIXES & PREFIXES PROMINENT IN MEDICAL TERMINOLOGY

	Definition	Example
A-, AN-	without	Anacidity (lack of acid)
AB-	away from	Abberation (away from normal growth)
AD-	toward	Adduction (bringing towards the body)
ADIP-	fat	Adipose (fat tissue)
ADEN-	gland	Adenoids (enlarged tonsils)
ANGI-	vessel	Angiogram (X-Ray of coronary arteries)
-ALGIA	pain	Arthralgia (pain in a joint)
ANA-	upwards	Anabasis (increasing severity of a disease)
ANTE-	before, in front of	Antenatal (occuring before birth)
ANTI-	against	Antifebrile (against fever)
APO-	separation from	Aponia (freedom from pain)
-AR	pertaining to	Lumbar (pertaining to the lower back)
ARTER-	artery	Arteriosclerosis (abnormal hardening of arterial walls)
ARTHRO-	joint	Arthritis (inflammation of a joint)
AUD-	hearing	Audiometry (measurement of hearing)
AUTO-	self	Auto-intoxication (poison generated within the body)

	Definition	Example
BI-	two	Binaural (pertaining to both ears)
BIO-	life	Biology (science of living organisms)
BLAST- **-BLAST**	embryo	Blastocyst (a stage of embryonic development)
CARDIO-	heart	Cardiovascular (pertaining to the heart and blood vessels)
CARP-	wrist	Carpals (bones of the wrist)
CIRCUM-	around	Circumduction (circular movement of a limb)
CO-	with	Coalesce (to grow together)
CYT-	cell	Cytoplasm (the protoplasm of a cell exclusive of the nucleus)
DE-	undoing	Degeneration (change from a higher to a lower form)
DI-	two	Diphasic (occuring in two stages)
DIA-	through	Diarthrosis (fully movable joint)
DIS-	lack of	Dis-ease (lack of comfort of mind and body)
DYS-	pain, difficulty	Dyspepsia (indigestion)
ECTO-	outer side	Ectoderm (outer layer of skin)
-ECTOMY	excision of	Appendectomy (surgical removal of the appendix)
EDEM-	swelling	Edema (abnormal accumulation of watery fluid in connective tissue)

	Definition	Example
-EMIA	blood	Leukemia (malignant disease of the blood-forming organs)
EN-	in, inside	Encapsulated (enclosed in a capsule)
ENDO-	within	Endocardium (lining membrane of heart)
EPI-	upon, over	Epidermis (top layer of skin)
EX-	out from	Excise (to remove by cutting out)
EXTRA-	outside of	Extramural (outside a tissue wall)
GASTR-	stomach	Gastritis (inflammation of the stomach)
-GENESIS	development, formation	Spermatogenesis (process by which sperm cells are formed)
-GLIA	glue	Neuroglia (cells that bind nerve tissue together)
-GRAM	something written	Myogram (recording of a muscular contraction)
HEM-	blood	Hemoglobin (coloring matter in the blood)
HEMI-	half	Hemiplegia (paralysis of one side of the body)
HEPAT-	liver	Hepatitis (inflammation of the liver)
HETERO-	different	Heteropsia (difference in vision between two eyes)
HOMEO-	same	Homeostasis (maintenance of a stable internal environment)

	Definition	Example
HYDRO-	water	Hydrology (science dealing with the properties of water)
HYPER-	over, above	Hyperextension (extreme or excessive extension of a limb or part)
HYPO-	under, below	Hypoglycemia (abnormally low sugar levels in the blood)
IMMUN-	free	Immunity (resistance to or freedom from a specific disease)
IN-	in, not	Insomnia (sleeplessness)
INFLAMM-	to heat up	Inflammation (condition characterized by reddened, warm, swollen tissues)
INFRA-	under, below	Infraspinatus (below the shoulder blade)
INTER-	between	Interphase (stage occurring between mitotic divisions of a cell.
INTRA-	within	Intracellular fluid (fluid within cells)
ISO-	equal	Isometric (maintaining the same measure or length)
-ITIS	inflammation of	Tonsilitis (inflammation of tonsils)
LOGY-	the study of	Physiology (study of body functions)
MACRO-	large	Macroblast (a very large red blood cell)
MAL-	bad, poor	Malnutrition (poor nutrition)

	Definition	Example
MEGAL-	enlarged	Megaloblastic Anemia (presence of large nucleated red blood cells)
MESO-	many	Mesodermal Cells (many types of cells)
-METER	measure	Calorimeter (instrument used to measure the caloric content of food)
MICRO-	small	Microplasia (dwarfism)
MONO-	one	Monosaccharide (a compound whose molecules consist of a single saccharide unit)
MOTO-	moving	Motor Neuron (neuron that stimulates a muscle to contract or gland to release a secretion)
MUT-	change	Mutation (a change in hereditary character)
MYELO-	spinal cord, bone marrow	Myelin (bone marrow)
Myo-	muscle	Myoma (tumor in muscle tissue)
NAS-	nose	Nasal (pertaining to the nose)
ORB-	circle	Orbital (portion of skull that encircles the eye)
PATHO-	disease	Pathogen (disease-causing agent)
-PLEGIA	paralysis	Paraplegia (paralysis of lower trunk and legs)
PLEUR-	rib	Pleural Membrane (membrane that encloses the lungs within the rib cage)

	Definition	Example
POLY-	many	Polycystic (containing many cysts)
POST-	behind, after	Post Mortem (after death)
PRE-	before, in front of	Prenatal (before birth)
PRO-	before or forward	Prognosis (forecast as to result of disease)
PSEUDO-	false	Pseudoangina (false angina)
PSYCHO-	mind	Psychoanalysis (mental examination)
REN-	kidney	Renal Cortex (outer region of the kidney)
RHINO-	nose	Rhinolith (calculus in nose)
SCHIZO-	splitting	Schizophrenia (mental disorder marked by loss of contact with reality)
SCLER-	tough, hard	Sclera (tough, outer protective layer of the eye)
-SCOPE **-SCOPY**	examining, to see	Pharyngoscope (instrument to examine pharynx)
SEMI-	half, partial	Semiconscious (partly conscious)
SENS-	feeling	Sensory Neuron (neuron that can be stimulated by a sensory receptor and conducts impulses into the brain or spinal cord)
-STASIS	slow, stop	Homeostasis (maintenance of stable internal environment)

	Definition	Example
-STOMY	formation of an opening in an organ by operation	Tracheostomy (formation of opening in trachea)
SUB-	under	Subcostal (situated beneath a rib)
SUPER- **SUPRA-**	above, beyond	Superficial (near surface)
SYN-	together	Synergetic (working together)
TACHY-	fast	Tachycardia (abnormally fast heartbeat)
THORAC-	chest	Thoracic (pertaining to the chest area)
THROMB-	clot	Thrombocyte (blood platelet that plays a roll in formation of blood clot)
-TOMY	cutting	Anatomy (study of structure involving the cutting or removing of body parts)
TRI-	three	Tricuspid (having three cusps)
TROPHIC-	development	Catastrophic (great disaster or misfortune)
TUBER-	swelling	Tuberculosis (disease characterized by formation of fibrous masses within lungs)
UNI-	one	Unilateral (affecting one side)
VAS-	vessel	Vasopressin (substance that causes blood vessel walls to contract)
VENTR-	belly	Ventral (a position toward the front of the body)

GLOSSARY OF BASIC MEDICAL TERMINOLOGY

ABCESS: A localized collection of pus caused by the body combating various bacteria. The symptoms of inflammation are redness, warmth, swelling, and pain.

ABDOMEN: The lower part of the trunk. Above, separated by the diaphragm, lies the thorax or chest; below lies the pelvis. The abdominal cavity contains the digestive organs, including the stomach and intestines, and the associated glands, the liver and pancreas.

ABDUCTION: A directional term indicating a movement of part of the body away from the midline. An example would be lifting your arm.

ABLATION: Removal of any part of the body by a surgical operation.

ABRASION: The rubbing off of the surface of the skin or mucous membrane due to injury. An effective form of treatment consists of thoroughly and immediately cleaning the wound with soap and water.

ACUPUNCTURE: A traditional Chinese method of treatment by puncture of a body part with needles. Its rationale is that disease is a manifestation of a disturbance of Yin and Yang (female and male) energy in the body, and that acupuncture brings this energy back into balance by the judicious stimulation or depression of the flow of energy in the various meridians.

ADDUCTION: A directional term indicating to move a part of the body toward the midline. An example would be lowering your arm towards your body.

ADHESION: The uniting together of structures which should normally be separate and freely movable. It results from acute or chronic inflammation.

ADJUST: To fix fast, an almost instantaneous concussion of forces designed to bring the area adjusted to a true or more effective relative position.

AGNESIA: Incomplete development or the failure of any part or organ of the body to develop normally.

ALIMENTARY CANAL: The passage along which food passes, extending from the mouth to the anus, including several accessory organs that release secretions into the canal. The alimentary canal includes the mouth, pharynx, esophagus, stomach, and the small and large intestines. The accessory organs include the salivary glands, liver, gallbladder, and pancreas.

ALLERGY: An individual's special sensitivity to certain foods, plants, animals, insect bites, etc.

ALLOPATHY: The methods used by regular practitioners of medicine and surgery. The term literally means "curing by inducing a different kind of action in the body."

AMINO-ACID: The components of protein broken down during digestion. These smaller molecules are absorbed and transported to the body cells in the blood. There are twenty to twenty-two amino acids. Eight are considered essential amino acids because they cannot be synthesized by the body and therefore must be present in the diet. The eight essential amino acids are isoleucine, leucine, lysine, methionine, phenylalanine, threonine, tryptophan, and valine.

AMPHETAMINES: A group of drugs closely related to adrenaline that act by stimulating the sympathetic nervous system.

ANATOMICAL POSITION: Face forward, arms down at the side with the thumbs out, and legs slightly spread apart.

ANATOMY: The science which deals with the structure or parts of an organism—how it's put together as related to the bodies of humans and animals.

ANEMIA: A condition characterized by inadequate red blood cells and/or hemoglobin in the blood.

ANGINA: Pain or a sensation of heavy pressure, tightening, or squeezing in the chest. The pain may also radiate to other parts, including the neck, jaw, throat, shoulder, or back. The condition is often associated to a decreased oxygen supply in the heart muscle, sometimes caused by the accumulation of solid materials inside the blood vessels.

ANKLYO: Relates to bending or crookedness, as well as to fusion or joining of specific structures.

ANOREXIA: A prolonged loss of appetite.

ANTERIOR: A directional term meaning "situated before or towards the front."

ATLAS: The first spinal vertebra, located in the neck.

AXIS: The second spinal vertebra.

AUTONOMIC NERVOUS SYSTEM: The portion of the nervous system that functions independently without conscious thought. It is concerned with regulating heart rate, blood pressure, breathing rate, body temperature, and other visceral functions. It has two main divisions, the sympathetic and parasympathetic.

BARBITURATES: A wide ranging group of sedative, hypnotic, and anaesthetic drugs.

BREAK: To separate into parts with suddenness or violence.

BRUISE: Injury of the deeper parts of the skin and underlying tissues, accompanied generally by outpouring of blood from damaged vessels, but not necessarily containing open wounds.

BULIMIA: An insatiable appetite often followed by stomach purging.

BURSITIS: Inflammation within a bursa (joint).

CALORIE: A unit of energy. The amount of heat required to raise one gram of water one degree centigrade in temperature, in normal use a kilocalorie.

CARBOHYDRATE: An organic substance containing hydrogen, carbon, and oxygen. Foods containing carbohydrates include sugars, starches, celluloses, and gums. When one of these foods is digested, it is converted into a simple kind of sugar and absorbed in this form.

CARDIOLOGY: A branch of medical science dealing with the heart and heart diseases.

CELLS: Microscopic particles that are the structural and functional unit of an organism.

CEREAL: Any plant similiar to grass, bearing an edible seed. The important cereals are wheat, oats, barley, maize, rice, and millet.

CERVICAL: Pertaining to the neck, specifically the first seven vertebrae.

CHIROPRACTIC: A philosophy, science, and art of things natural; a system of adjusting the segments of the spinal column by hand only, for the correction of the cause of dis-ease. (From Volume 14, *Chiropractic Text Book*, pages xxx-xxxiii, B.J. Palmer, 1927).

CHOLESTEROL: A lipid or fat, produced by body cells used in the synthesis of steriod hormones, excreted into the bile. Excessive amounts of cholesterol in the body can result in plaqueing of the arteries, which contributes to hardening of the arteries.

CHROMOSOMES: Rod-shaped bodies found in the nucleus of every cell in the body. They contain the genes, or hereditary elements, which establish the characteristics of an individual.

CIRCUMDUCTION: A directional term meaning to move a part of the body so that its end follows a circular path. An example would be moving the finger in a circular motion without moving the hand.

COCCYX: The end of the vertebral (spinal) column beyond the sacrum.

COMPENSATION: The counterbalancing of some defect of structure or function by some other special bodily development. The body possesses remarkable powers of adapting itself to even serious defects, so that disability due to these may diminish over time.

CONCUSSION: The bruising of part of the brain, usually resulting from a blow to the head.

CONSTITUTION: The general condition of the body, especially with reference to its susceptibility to certain diseases.

CONVALESCENCE: The condition a person passes through after suffering from an acute disease and before complete health and strength are regained.

CONVULSIONS: Rapidly alternating contractions and relaxations of the muscles, causing irregular movements of the limbs or body generally, and usually accompanied by unconsciousness.

COORDINATION: The governing power exercised by the brain as a whole, or by certain centers in the nervous system, to make muscles contract in harmony and for the internal organs and the body as a whole to function together in harmony.

CRANIUM: The part of the skull enclosing the brain, as distinguished from the face.

CYTOLOGY: A branch of medical science dealing with the structure, function, and diseases of cells.

DELIRIUM: A state of altered consciousness in which an irregular discharge of nervous energy goes on, causing incoherent speech, delusions, and poorly regulated muscular action.

DERMATOLOGY: A branch of medical science dealing with the study of the skin and its diseases.

DETOXIFICATION: Reduction or removal of toxic substances.

DEXTRO: A directional term referring to the right.

DIAGNOSIS: The art of distinguishing one disease from another.

DIAPHRAGM: The muscular partition which separates the cavity of the abdomen from that of the thoracic region or chest area. The diaphragm assists the breathing process by increasing and decreasing the size of the thoracic cavity.

DIATHERMY: A process by which electric currents can be passed into the deeper parts of the body to produce internal warmth and relieve pain; or by using powerful currents, to destroy tumors and diseased parts bloodlessly.

DISCS: Fibrocartilage located between the vertebra of the spinal column. They are designed to act as shock absorbers for the spine and allow painless movement of the individual vertebra, giving the body the ability to have motion.

DISLOCATION: The displacement of one or more bones at a joint.

DISTAL: A directional term meaning "further away from the point of origin."

DNA: Deoxyribonucleic acid. Molecules that store information in the manner of a molecular code. This information tells cell parts how to construct specific protein molecules. Many of these proteins act as enzymes and are responsible for all of the metabolic reactions that occur in cells. DNA molecules have the unique ability to duplicate themselves prior to cell reproduction. Each newly formed cell receives an exact copy of the instructions for carrying on vital life processes.

DORSAL: A directional term meaning "behind."

DORSIFLEXION: Flexing the foot at the ankle by bending the foot upward.

ELEVATION: Raising a part of the body.

ENDOCRINOLOGY: A branch of medical science dealing with hormone-secreting glands and their diseases.

EPIDEMIOLOGY: A branch of medical science dealing with infectious diseases, their distribution, and control.

ETIOLOGY: A branch of medical science dealing with the causes of disease.

EUTHANASIA: The procuring of an easy and painless death.

EVERSION: Turning the foot so the sole is outward.

EXTENSION: A directional term indicating the action of straightening parts at a joint so that the angle between them is increased and the parts move further apart, such as straightening the leg at the knee.

FAINTING: The temporary loss of consciousness.

FASCIA: Sheets or bands of fibrous tissue which enclose a muscle.

FLEXION: A directional term indicating bending parts at a joint so that the angle between them is increased and the parts move closer together, such as bending the leg at the knee.

FORAMEN MAGNUM: The opening in the occipital bone of the skull, through which the spinal cord passes.

FRACTURE: A break in a bone, usually produced by violent trauma.

GASTRIC: Related to the stomach.

GASTROENTEROLOGY: A branch of medical science dealing with the stomach, intestines, and the diseases that affect them.

GENES: A portion of a DNA molecule that contains the information needed to synthesize an enzyme. Genes are the biological units of heredity.

GENETICS: The study of the mechanisms by which characteristics are passed from parents to offspring, or the study of heredity.

GERIATRICS: A branch of medical science dealing with diseases associated with old age.

GERONTOLOGY: A branch of medical science involving the study of the ageing process and problems of elderly persons.

GLUTEAL: The region of the buttocks and the structures situated in it, such as the gluteal muscles, arteries, and nerves.

GYNECOLOGY: A branch of medical science dealing with the female reproductive system and its diseases.

HELIOTHERAPY: The treatment of disease by exposing the body to the sun's rays.

HEMATOLOGY: A branch of medical science dealing with the blood and its diseases.

HEREDITY: The principle on which various characteristics are transmitted from parents to offspring in the form of genetic information.

HERNIA: The protusion of any organ or part of an organ into or through the wall of the cavity which contains it.

HISTOLOGY: A branch of medical science dealing with the structure, function, and diseases of tissues.

HOMEOPATHY: A system of medicine based upon the theory that diseases are curable by those drugs which produce effects on the body similar to symptoms caused by the disease. In administering drugs, the theory is held that their effect is increased by giving them to an extreme degree.

HOMEOSTASIS: A state of equilibrium in which the internal environment of the body remains relatively constant.

HYPEREXTENSION: Excessive extension of the parts at a joint beyond a normal anatomical range of motion.

IATROGENIC: From the roots *iatro* meaning "physician" and *genic,* meaning "produced by." Generally refers to diseases caused as a side effect of taking drugs administered by a doctor.

IDIOPATHIC: Diseases whose cause is unknown.

ILIUM: The largest and uppermost portion of the coxal or hip bone.

IMMUNITY: A principle by virtue of which the body is protected from the invasion of certain diseases or the action of certain poisons.

IMPACTION: A condition in which two things are firmly lodged together.

INFECTION: A condition caused by the presence of invading microorganisms.

INFERIOR: A directional term meaning "below."

INVERSION: Turning the foot so the sole is inward.

ISCHIUM: The lowest portion of the hip bone which supports the weight of the body when a person is sitting.

KINESIOLOGY: A branch of medical science dealing with the study of the principles of mechanics and anatomy in relation to human movement.

KYPHOSIS: Abnormally increased convexity (forward curving) in the curvature of the thoracic spine as viewed from the side. Also know as humpback or hunchback.

LAMINECTOMY: Surgical removal of the posterior arch of a vertebra, usually to relieve the symptoms of a ruptured intervertebral disc.

LATERAL: A directional term meaning "away from the midline or closer to the side."

LORDOSIS: Relating to the curving of the spine forward. This occurs in the cervical and lumbar regions of the spine. Lordosis can also denote abnormal curvature, especially in the lumbar region.

LUMBAR: Relating to the vertebrae between the thoracic vertebrae and the sacrum, commonly called the lower back.

LUMBAGO: A painful ailment affecting the lower part of the back.

LUXATION: To throw out of place or out of joint, as in a dislocation.

LYMPH: The fluid which circulates in the lymphatic vessels of the body. The lymphatic system provides pathways through which tissue fluids can be transported as lymph from the interstitial spaces located between cells, other than blood cells, to veins. This lymph empties into the blood through either the thoracic duct or the right lymphatic duct.

MEDIAL: A directional term meaning "midline down the center." Speaking lengthwise, medial is nearer the midline.

MEDICINE: The science and art dealing with the maintenance of health and the prevention, alleviation, or cure of disease.

MIGRAINE: Recurring intense headaches.

NATUROPATHY: A system of treatment of disease emphasizing assistance to nature and including the use of natural medicinal substances and physical means.

NERVES: Nerves, or nerve cells called neurons, comprise the basic components of the nervous system. The nervous system acts primarily in the coordination of the organs and systems of the body. It senses the environment, interprets what is going on, then coordinates the reaction. This is done in four ways: converting stimulus into nerve impulses, interpreting the meaning of the impulses, sorting out impulses that are most important by prioritizing the stimulus, sending out impulses to the effectors or the parts of the body that cause you to react such as muscles or glands.

Nerves vary much in size. The sciatic nerve, located in the muscles on the back of the thigh, is the largest nerve in the body, being the thickness of a lead pencil or more. Other nerves are smaller in size, (down to 2 to 15 microns). A nerve such as the sciatic, possesses a strong, outer fibrous sheath, called the epineurium, within which lie bundles of nerve-fibers, divided from one another by partitions of fibrous tissue, in which run blood vessels that nourish the nerve. Each of these bundles is surrounded by its own sheath, known as the perineurium, and within the bundle fine partitions of fibrous tissue, known as endoneurium, divide up the bundle into groups of fibers.

NEUROLOGY: A branch of medical science dealing with the nervous system and its diseases.

NEUROTIC: A general term of indefinite meaning applied to a person of nervous temperament, whose actions are largely determined by emotions or instincts rather than by reason.

OBESITY: A condition of the body characterized by over accumulation of fat under the skin and around certain internal organs. Also known as corpulence.

ONCOLOGY: A branch of medical science dealing with tumors of the body.

OPTHALMOLOGY: A branch of medical science dealing with the eye and its diseases.

ORTHOPEDICS: A branch of medical science dealing with the muscular and skeletal systems and their problems.

OSTEOPATHY: A system of healing in which diseases are treated by manipulating bones and other parts with the idea of thereby restoring functions in bodily mechanisms that have become deranged.

OTORHINOLARYNGOLOGY: A branch of medical science dealing with the ear, nose, and throat, and their diseases.

PALLIATIVE: The treatment of incurable diseases, in which the aim is to mitigate the sufferings of the patient, not to effect a cure.

PALPATION: The art of feeling with the hand or a method of examining the surface of the body and the size, shape, and movements of the internal organs by laying the fingers of the hand upon the skin.

PALPITATION: A condition in which the heart beats forcibly or irregularly and the person becomes conscious of its action.

PANACEA: A remedy for all diseases, or indicating a remedy which benefits many different diseases.

PARALYSIS: Loss of muscular power due to interference with the nervous system. Also called palsy.

PARANOIA: A form of fixed delusional insanity in which the delusions, usually of persecution, have an important bearing upon the person's actions. Heredity can be a factor and in marked cases, restraint is often necessary to prevent criminal acts.

PATHOGENIC: Disease producing. Applies to bacteria and other substances capable of causing disease.

PATHOLOGY: A branch of medical science dealing with the causes of and changes produced in the body by disease.

PEDIATRICS: A branch of medical science dealing with children and their diseases.

PELVIS: The part of the skeleton which is made up of hip bones, one on each side, and the sacrum and coccyx behind. It connects the lower limbs with the spine. Each hip bone is composed of three originally separate bones firmly fused together in the adult pelvis, the ilium, the ischium, with a rounded part below, the tuberosity, upon which the body rests in sitting; and the pubis in front.

PERCUSSION: An aid to diagnosis, practiced by striking the body with the fingers or with an instrument known as a plessor in such a way as to make it give out a note. According to the degree of dullness or resonance of the note, an opinion can be formed as to the state of consolidation of air-containing organs, the presence of abnormal cavities in organs, and the dimensions of solid and air-containing organs.

PHARMACOLOGY: A branch of medical science dealing with knowledge of the action of drugs.

PHYSIOLOGY: A branch of medical science dealing with the functions of different organs and the changes that the whole body undergoes in the course of the treatment of disease. Also known as physical medicine.

PHYSIOTHERAPY: A form of treatment involving the use of physical measures, such as exercise, heat, and massage in the treatment of disease. Also known as physical medicine.

PLACEBO: An inactive substance given to a patient, not because it will have any definite action but because the patient will not be satisfied without some active treatment. Also used as a control mechanism in experiments.

PLANTAR FLEXION: Extending the foot at the ankle by bending the foot downward.

POSTERIOR: A directional term referring to being situated behind.

PROGNOSIS: A forecast as to the probable result of an illness or disease, particularly with regard to the prospect of recovery, based upon the nature and symptoms of the case.

PRONATION: Turning the hand so the palm is downward.

PROTEIN: Members of a group of non-crystallizable nitrogenous substances widely distributed in the animal and vegetable kingdoms and forming the characteristic materials of their tissues and fluids. They are essentially combinations of amino-acids. They are dissolved by various chemical substances.

Proteins constitute an essential part of the diet as a source of energy and for the replacement of protein lost in the wear and tear of daily life. Their essential constituent is the nitrogen they contain. To be absorbed or digested, proteins have to be broken down into their constituent amino-acids. The adult human body can maintain nitrogenous equilibrium on a mixture of eight amino-acids, known as the essential amino-acids.

PROXIMAL: A directional term referring to the part of the body that is closer to a point of attachment or to the trunk of the body.

PROTRACTION: Moving a part of the body forward.

PSYCHIATRY: A branch of medical science dealing with the mind and its disorders.

PUBIS: The bone that forms the front part of the pelvis. The pubic bones of opposite sides meet in the symphsis and protect the bladder from the front.

RADIOLOGY: A branch of medical science dealing with X-rays and radioactive substances and their uses in the diagnosis and treatment of diseases.

REHABILITATION: The restoration to health and working capacity of a person mentally or physically incapacitated.

RESOLUTION: Applies to infective processes, indicating a natural subsidence of inflammation without the formation of pus. Thus a pneumonic lung is said to achieve resolution when the material exuded into it is absorbed into the blood and lymph so that recovery takes place naturally.

RESPIRATION: Related to the breathing action of the lungs, the process in which air passes into and out of the lungs, with the object of allowing the blood to absorb oxygen and to give off carbon dioxide and water. Respiration occurs eighteen times a minute in a healthy adult at rest.

RETRACTION: Moving a part of the body backward.

RETRO: A directional term meaning behind, in back of.

ROTATION: A directional term referring to moving a part of the body around an axis, such as twisting the head from side to side.

SACRUM: A portion of the spinal column near its lower end. The sacrum consists of five vertebrae fused together to form a broad triangular bone which lies between the two hip bones and forms the back wall of the pelvis.

SAGITTAL: A directional term applied to a structure or section running from front to back in the body.

SANITATION: The science which aims at the prevention of disease through cleanliness, enlisting the knowledge of medicine, bacteriology, and engineering.

SCAPULA: The scientific name for the shoulder blade.

SCAR: A healed wound, ulcer, or breach of tissue. A scar consists essentially of fibrous tissue covered by an imperfect formation of the skin. The fibrous tissue is produced by the connective tissue corpuscles that wander into the wound in the course of its repair and is at first delicate in texture and richly provided with blood vessels. Accordingly, a scar at first is soft and has a redder tint then that of the surounding skin. Gradually this fibrous tissue contracts, becomes more dense, and loses its blood vessels, so that an old scar is hard and white.

SCIATICA: Pain along the course of the sciatic nerve. It is often acompanied by pain in the back. Generally, the pain is felt in the buttocks, the back of the thigh and the outside and front of the leg, sometimes extending on to the top of the foot. In other cases the pain is felt in the buttocks, the back of the thigh and the calf, and then along the outer border of the foot towards the little toe.

SCOLIOSIS: Curvature of the spine, consisting partly of a bend to one side, partly of a rotary twist. It may result from disease of the spine. In children, especially, it can occur from poor posture habits. It also arises from disease affecting one side of the chest, such as chronic pleurisy or tuberculosis.

SEPSIS: Poisoning by the products of putrefaction. This process is set up by the growth of micro-organisms in the body. The general symptoms which accompany it are those of inflammation.

SINISTRO: A directional term referring to the left.

SKELETON: The comprehensive term applied to the hard structures that support or protect the softer tissues of the body. The skeleton is divided into two main portions: the axial skeleton and the appendicular skeleton. The axial skeleton contains the bony and cartilaginous parts that support and protect the organs of the head, neck, and trunk. This includes the skull, hyoid bone, vertebral column, and thoracic cage. The appendicular skeleton consists of the bones of the limbs and those that anchor them to the axial skeleton. This includes the pectoral girdle, (shoulder blade and collarbone) pelvic girdle, and upper and lower limbs which make up the arms and legs.

SKULL: Twenty-two flat and irregularly shaped bones which protect the brain and form the face comprise the skull. In early life the brain and organs of special sense are enclosed in a case which is formed partly of cartilage, partly of a fibrous membrane. The transformation into bone, ossification, begins early in life, and the bone gradually spreads outwards from each of these centers.

The bones are fastened to one another by sutures, joints in which each edge is locked with the edges of neighboring bones by exactly fitting projections and depressions, resembling a complicated mortise-work. Occasionally small bones develop in the sutures, these extra bones being known as sutural or wormian bones.

The skull consists of two distinct parts: the cranium, which encloses the brain and consists of eight bones, and the face, which forms a bony framework for the eyes, nose, and mouth, and is composed of fourteen bones. These two parts can be detached from one another. The lower jaw is connected with the base of the cranium by a movable joint on each side.

The interior of the cranium is molded so as to form a support for the brain. Its base is divided by bony ridges into three fossa, which support the frontal lobes and the cerebellum. The inner surface of the bone shows grooves and hollows corresponding to the convolutions and blood vessels of the brain. The bones, especially on the base of the skull, are pierced by many small canals (foramina) which transmit nerves and blood vessels. Of these, the largest is the foramen magnum, through which the medulla oblongata and the spinal cord connect.

SLIPPED DISC: Also known as a prolapsed intervertebral disc. A misnomer. Discs don't slip. They rupture (See Chapter 10). The spinal column is built up of a series of bones, known as vertebrae, placed one upon the other. Between these vertebrae lay a series of thick discs of fibro-cartilage known as intervertebral discs. Each disc consists of an outer portion, the annulus fibrosis, and an inner core, the nucleus pulposis.

The function of the discs is to give flexibility and resiliency to the spinal column and to act as buffers against undue jarring, acting as efficient shock absorbers. They may, however, prolapse, or protrude, between the two adjacent vertebrae. If this happens they press on the neighboring spinal nerve and cause pain. The most common sites of protrusion, or prolapse, are between the last two lumbar vertebrae and between the last lumbar vertebra and the sacrum. This means that the pain occurs in the back, causing lumbago, or along the course of the sciatic nerve, causing sciatica.

SPASM: An involuntary, and in severe cases, painful contraction of a muscle or of a hollow organ with a muscular wall. Spasm may be due to affections in the muscle where the spasm takes place, or it may originate in some disturbance of that part of the nervous system which controls the spasmodically acting muscles.

SPINAL COLUMN: The spinal column is the rigid foundation which supports the upper parts of the body as well as protecting the spinal cord and the nerves that exit it. The spinal column contains vertebrae, bones that are capable of a slight degree of turning and movement. The possession of a spinal cord supported by a vertebral column distinguishes the higher animals from the lower types, giving them the general name of vertebrates. Of the vertebrates, man alone stands absolutely erect, and this erect carriage of the body gives to the skull and vertebral column certain distinctive characteristics.

The spinal column is about 28 inches (70cm) in length, and varies little in fully grown persons. The number of vertebrae is thirty-three in children, although in adult life five of these fuse together to form the sacrum, and the lowest four unite in the coccyx, reducing the number of separate bones to twenty-four. There are seven cervical vertebrae comprising the neck, twelve thoracic or dorsal vertebrea with ribs attached comprising the thoracic region, and five lumbar vertebrae contained in the lower spine.

Although the vertebrae in each of these regions have distinguishing features, all are of similar construction. Each has a thick, rounded, bony part in front, known as the body, and these bodies form the main thickness of the column. Behind the body of each is a ring of bone, the neural ring. These rings,placed one above another, form the bony canal which holds the spinal cord. From each side of the ring a short projection of bone known as the transverse process stands out, and from the back of the ring a larger process, the spinous process, projects. These processes give attachment to the strong ligaments and muscles which unite, support, and bend the column. The spinous processes can be seen or felt beneath the skin of the back. The spinous process of the seventh cervical vertebra, is especially large and forms a distinct bony prominence where the neck joins the back.

Between the bodies of the vertebrae is a series of thick discs of fibro-cartilage known as intervertebral discs. Each disc consists of an outer portion, known as the annulus fibrosus, and an inner core, known as the nucleus pulposus. These twenty-three discs give the spinal column a great deal of resiliency and power of diminishing the effect of forces communicated through the feet or head. There is also a small joint at each side upon the ring of the vertebra so that each vertebra comes in contact with the one above and the one beneath in three places.

The first and second cervical vertebrae are special modifications. The first vertebra, the atlas, is devoid of a body, but has a specially large and strong ring with two hollows, upon which the skull rests, thus permitting nodding movements. The second vertebra, the axis, has a pivot upon its body which fits into the first vertebra and thus permits free rotation of the head from side to side.

An important feature of the spinal column, and one especially marked in human beings, is the presence of the curves from back to front. The cervical curvature in the neck and the lumbar curvature in the lower back are convex anteriorly while the thoracic and pelvic curvatures are concave anteriorly. The effect of the thoracic and pelvic curves is to increase the size of the cavities of the chest and pelvis, while the compensating curves of the neck and lower back serve to keep the general axis of the spinal column in a vertical line. The curves have also an action very similar to that of the springs of a vehicle in minimizing jolting and jarring of the internal organs.

The neural rings placed one above another form a canal, which is wide in the neck, smaller and almost round in the dorsal region, and wide again in the lumbar vertebrae. This canal holds the spinal cord. The nerves that issue from the cord exit from the canal through openings between the vertebrae on the upper and lower margins of each ring.

SPINAL CORD: The spinal cord is the lower portion of the central nervous system which is situated within the spinal column. Above, it forms the direct continuation of the medulla oblongata. This part of the brain changes its name to the spinal cord at the foramen magnum, the large opening in the base of the skull through which it passes into the spinal canal. Below, the spinal cord extends to about the upper border of the second lumbar vertebra, where it tapers off into descending nerves that form a structure known as the cauda equina, which is shaped similar to a horse's tail.

The spinal cord is considerably shorter than the spinal column, being only 15 to 18 inches (37 to 45 cm) in length and weighing around 30 grams. In its course from the base of the skull to lumbar region the cord gives off thirty-one nerves on each side, each of which arises by an anterior and a posterior root that join before the nerve emerges from the spinal canal.

The spinal cord is cylindrical in shape, about the thickness of the little finger, and slightly flattened from front to back. It has two slightly enlarged portions, one in the lower part of the neck, the other at the last dorsal vertebra, and from these enlargements extend the nerves that pass to the upper and lower limbs. The spinal cord, like the brain, is surrounded by three membranes, the dura mater, arachnoid mater, and pia mater, from the outside to the inside.

The spinal cord is a receiver and originator of nerve impulses, and in part merely a conductor of such impulses along fibers which pass through it to and from the brain.

Diseases and injuries of the spinal cord are considered together because the chief danger of interference with the spinal column lies in the risk of injury to the spinal cord and nerves. The seriousness of most diseases affecting the spine is measured by their tendency to interfere with the spinal cord. The following are some of the more common diseases affecting the spinal cord and spinal column.

Sprains of the back due to a twist and leading to tearing of muscles and ligaments may be responsible for long-continued pain and even paralysis, probably due to injury of the spinal nerves.

Lateral curvature of the spine (scoliosis) consists chiefly in a bending of the spine over to one side. This is accompanied by a certain amount of twisting of the vertebrae around their vertical axis. The shape of the chest becomes markedly altered, the ribs on one side projecting behind at their angles and causing the shoulder blade to be very prominent, while on the other side the chest is flattened.

Backward curvature of the spine (kyphosis), commonly referred to as humpback, may be due to various causes. One cause is tuberculosis of the spine. This results in destruction and collapse of one or more vertebrae with posterior angulation of the spine. Other causes are what is known as compression fracture of the spine following an accident, spondylitis, rickets, or conditions which cause decalcification or softening of the bones, such as osteomalacia. The round shoulders of the adolescent, due to faulty posture and lack of exercise, is a form of more generalized kyphosis.

Compression of the spinal cord may be caused suddenly by a severe crush or blow upon the back, which produces a fracture of the spine with displacement of the fragments.

Spondylitis, or inflammation of the vertebrae of the spine, may occur at any age, but is a disease predominantly of young men between the ages of twenty and forty. Unless treated in the early stages, it tends to run an inexorable course, ultimately leading to complete fixation of the spine as result of bony ankylosis between the vertebrae.

Spondylolisthesis is a congenital defect of the spine, usually affecting the fifth lumbar vertebra. This results in slipping forward of the affected vertebra, which induces backache.

Meningitis is a term applied to inflammation affecting the membranes of the brain (cerebral meningitis) or spinal cord (spinal meningitis) or both. Either the dura or the pia-arachnoid may be inflamed. In the former case, the condition is known as pachymeningitis; in the later, leptomeningitis.

Myelitis, or inflammation situated in the spinal cord itself, may be of an acute or chronic nature and gives rise to symptoms much resembling those of compression, though unaccompanied by pain. A special form of myelitis is poliomyelitis, which affects only the grey matter of the cord.

Sclerosis is a chronic condition of the cord in which certain parts become increasingly hard through disappearance of the white nerve fibers and are replaced by an overgrowth of the connective tissue of the cord. This change may be due to various causes, and the symptoms which it produces depend mainly upon the particular tracts of fibers that are affected. Sclerosis in the posterior part of the cord, for example, produces the disease known as locomotor ataxia. Multiple sclerosis, in which the degenerated patches are scattered through the nervous system, affects mainly the lateral portions of the cord.

STENOSIS: A condition of unnatural narrowing in any passage or orifice of the body.

SUBLUXATION: A vertebra out of position in relationship to the one above or below it. As a result, pressure is placed on the nerves that exit the spinal column between the vertebrae. When there is a subluxation, the following four conditions occur: The spine is out of alignment, is out of its normal range of motion, has a fixation between two or more vertebrae, and is causing interference to the nerve impulses exiting between the vertebrae.

SUPERIOR: A directional term meaning "situated above."

SUPINATION: Turning the hand so the palm is upward.

SYMPATHETIC NERVOUS SYSTEM: Part of the autonomic nervous system consisting of scattered collections of grey matter known as ganglia, united by an irregular network of nerve fibers. Those portions where the ganglia are placed most closely and where the network of fibers is especially dense are known as plexuses. The chief part of the sympathetic system consists of two ganglionated cords that run through the neck, chest, and abdomen, lying close in front of the spine.

THERAPEUTICS: A general name applied to the science and art of healing.

THERAPY: The treatment of disease.

THORACIC: Of, relating to, located within, or involving the thorax or chest.

TORTICOLLIS: A condition in which the head is twisted to one side. It may be caused by the contraction of a scar, such as that resulting from a burn, or by paralysis of some of the muscles. In the great majority of cases it is a spasmodic condition due to excessive contraction of certain muscles. Also know as wry-neck.

TOXICOLOGY: A branch of medical science dealing with poisions and their effect on the body.

TRAUMA: Disorders due to wounds or injuries.

TREMOR: A very slight type of jerking spasm. Tremors may be seen in projecting parts like the hands, head, and tongue, or they may involve muscles or even the individual fibers of a muscle. They are of various grades of subtlety.

TUMOR: Literally, any swelling, but generally not including passing swellings caused by acute inflammation. The collections of diseased material arising in the course of chronic inflammation, like tuberculosis, syphilis, and leprosy, may or may not be classed as tumors, according to their size and appearance.

Tumors are divided into two classifications. One type is simple or benign, growing slowly at one spot, pressing neighboring parts aside but not invading them, not recurring after removal, and having little tendency to ulcerate. The other type is called malignant, spreading quickly from point to point, invading and destroying surrounding tissues, tending to recur after apparently complete removal, and being liable to ulcerate. This distinction dates back to the days of Hippocrates, who gave to gnawing tumors the name of carcinoma.

UROLOGY: A branch of medical science dealing with disorders and diseases of the kidneys, ureters, bladder, prostate, and urethra.

VEGETARIANISM: The principle of subsisting on a diet which contains no meat. Variations on such a diet may include milk, cheese and eggs.

VERTEBRA: One of the thirty-three irregularly shaped bones that together form the vertebral column (see spinal column.)

VITAMINS: Groups of substances which exist in minute quantities in natural foods and which are necessary to normal nutrition, especially in connection with growth and development. Several of them have now been synthesized. When they are absent from food, defective growth takes place in children, and in adults various diseases arise. Persistant deprivation of one or more vitamins can lead to a state of lowered general health.

WHIPLASH INJURY: Injury resulting from a sudden sharp whipping movement of the neck and head (as in a passenger in a vehicle that is struck head on or from the rear).

WOUNDS: A breach suddenly produced in the tissues of the body by direct violence. An extensive injury of the deeper parts without corresponding injury of the surface is known as a bruise or contusion.

NOTES

[1] (p.4) The written works of Hippocrates were most likely added to by other physicians of that time who held similar philosophical viewpoints. Hippocrates' own words are often paraphrased in quotations. Also attributed to him is the following: "One should first get a knowledge of the structure of the spine, for this is also requisite for many diseases" (Petersen 77).

[2] (p.18) From 1906 to 1961 B.J. Palmer published over forty books pertaining to chiropractic and health care in general. His publication, *Chiropractic Philosophy: Booklet #1* contains a compilation of philosophical writings found in those books.

[3] (p.26) I cannot overemphasize that a major issue confronting health care in this country is that we too often treat only the symptoms of disease and not the cause or causes behind them.

Statistics continually point out how lifestyle factors (diet, exercise, habits, etc.) contribute to the costs of health care. *The Sports Medicine Fitness Course* from which I cite this reference explains how individuals can have the greatest effect over their health. The result is providing ourselves with a better quality of life, along with reducing the tremendous economic burden that health care places on society. David Nieman, the author, states:

> It has been estimated that over 50% of all medical expenditures of total medical costs reflect an adverse personal lifestyle—particularly the abuse of cigarettes and alcohol. In a one-year project with three large groups involving instruction on self-care, total medical visits declined 17% and visits to doctors' offices for minor illnesses fell 35%. According to Vickery of the Center for Corporate Health Promotion, 20-70% of doctor's visits are unnecessary, and fewer than 10% of all visits to emergency rooms are critical enough to require immediate attention (20).

[4] (p.33) The major reason for taking care of your spine is to maintain the proper functioning of your nervous system. Nerve root impingement can result from improper juxtaposition of two or more vertebrae, damage of the intervertebral disc, trauma or even stress due to poor posture and lifting habits. In the book *Backache at Work*, M. Laurens Rowe further defines improper juxtaposition:

> Since one vertebra is attached to the next by a three point suspension system, narrowing of the disc space forces alterations in the two facet joints. More weight falls upon them and the articular cartilage with which their surfaces are faced gradually thins out and degenerates with narrowing of the joint spaces.... The lower back corner of the vertebra sags into the nerve root port hole from the front, and the tip of the articular process of the lower vertebra intrudes from behind. With the exit port constricted in both vertical and horizontal dimensions and distorted in contour, there is loss of the margin of safety for the nerve root.... As the disc casing becomes further thinned and weakened, the packing material may bulge outwards into the exit port creating pressure on the nerve root, or the casing may suddenly rupture completely, allowing a blowout of the packing material which compresses the nerve root in its shrunken and deformed port hole.... Failure of the disc allows abnormal motion to occur between vertebrae and, as it goes flat, throws heavy stress on the facet joints causing them to sublux and ultimately degenerate. The spatial integrity of the exit port holes for the nerve roots is violated (32-34).

[5] (p.36) Dr. Pettibon has been a practicing chiropractor for over thirty years. By realizing that the construction of the human spine is similar to that of a bridge, Pettibon has developed methods to analyze the condition and configuration of the spine.

His techniques establish a basis for understanding and communicating the condition of a patient's spine and the adjusting techniques employed. His methods are practiced throughout the chiropractic profession. I have attended his programs in spinal bio-mechanics, X-ray procedure and analysis, and adjusting techniques. In addition to many articles published in chiropractic journals, he has written several books, including one involving use of X-ray as pertaining to the spine called *True Plane Spinography*. This book explains the viewing of the spine as a three dimensional object.

[6] (p.41) That the health of the body is influenced by the condition of the spinal column and the capacity of the nervous system itself is indisputable. What is fascinating is the tremendous insight that many of the pioneers such as D.D. Palmer had in the field of health care. In his book *The Chiropractor's Adjustor*, Palmer relates how important the nervous system is in regards to man's ability to interact with his environment. He states:

> By the nervous system we become cognizant of our surroundings, because of impressions made upon their peripheral endings. It is through them that we regard the outer world. By the knowledge thus derived, we are able to adapt ourselves to our environment, receive sensations and direct motions (79).

[7] (p. 49) In the book *The Chiropractic Theories*, Robert A. Leach DC, reviews current scientific data regarding the chiropractic profession. As science further explores the brain and nervous system, findings bear out the Palmers' theories regarding function of the nervous system in relation to the structure of the body, particularly the exacting position of spinal vertebrae. The author explains the intervertebral foramen and nerve root passing out from it:

> The nerve roots and their sheaths occupy between 35% and 50% of the total cross sectional area of the intervertebral foramen, with the former figure pertaining especially to the dorsal foramina. The remaining 50% to 65% of the foramen contains loose areolar connective and adipose tissue with the spinal artery, numerous veins, lymphatics, and the recurrent meningeal nerve. These latter contents provide the nerve roots with an ample cushion from the periosteal boundaries of the foramen (51).

[8] (p.49) D.D. Palmer's basic premise was that when a vertebra was out of place, it could press on the adjacent spinal nerve and in the process, increase or decrease the flow of nerve energy carried by that particular spinal nerve. The pages listed cite numerous studies documenting intervertebral subluxations as a cause of spinal nerve root compression.

Since it has been determined that subluxations of the spinal column can compress nerve roots causing irritation and disease, it is vital that research be continued to learn exactly what occurs to the structure and function of the human body as a result of this condition.

[9] (p.57) M. Laurens Rowe MD, in his book *Backache at Work*, explains costs and problems associated with back injuries and spinal problems. The specific reference states:

> The National Safety Council estimates that 20% of all occupational injuries involve the back and this figure is in general agreement with experience in the nine states whose Workers' Compensation Boards or Commissions publish detailed statistics (6).

In the introduction the author states:

> Disability attributed to low back pain is industry's most expensive medical problem. Workers' Compensation costs for back cases far exceed those for other industrial injuries. Low back disability is among the leading causes of absence from work due to illness qualifying for sickness benefits (1).

[10] (p.59) In his book *Old Dad Chiro*, Vern Gielow details the life and times of D.D. Palmer, the Father of Chiropractic. The author worked for the Palmer College of Chiropractic for over twenty years and prior to that was involved in radio broadcasting with Palmer's son, B.J. Gielow's sources include Palmer's books and personal journal. Medical philosophies of Palmer's time are presented, as well as historical information pertinent to the Davenport area where Palmer was a resident and formed the first chiropractic school.

[11] (p.64) *The Ethics of Chiropractic*, by Bernard L. CiRullo Jr. DC, details the ethics of health care, especially as related to chiropractic. The author was a student of B.J. Palmer and, a graduate of the Palmer School (College) of Chiropractic. Palmer personally instructed Dr. CiRullo to learn from the practice of many chiropractors. Subsequently, he is the only person who has worked with at least one graduate of the college every ten years since the inception of chiropractic in 1895. CiRullo has spent years researching what chiropractic is, what it is not, and what services chiropractors can technically and legally render.

[12] (p.83) Because the word *subluxation* is used in instances other than intervertebral subluxations, experts in orthopedics, chiropractic, and roentgenology (X-ray) tend to differ on the characteristics and meaning of the word. In his book *The Chiropractic Theories*, Robert A. Leach DC states:

> Perhaps the most acknowledged definition in chiropractic today was presented at the National Institutes for Neurological Diseases and Stroke (now the National Institute of Neurological and Communicative Disorders and Stroke, NINCDS) workshop on spinal manipulative therapy: A subluxation is the alteration of the normal dynamics, anatomical or physiological relationship of contiguous articular structures (16,17).

[13] (p.105) Laurens M. Lowe MD says in his book *Backache at Work*:

> Anything which imbalances the trunk and thereby requires more muscular effort to maintain the upright position constitutes a functional abnormality.... The simplest example of a functional abnormality is pregnancy, which is often associated with low back pain. Here, an unaccustomed weight located forward of the center of gravity must be counterbalanced by muscular contraction. In addition, the load tilts the pelvis forward increasing the angle of take-off of the spine and, consequently, of the compensatory lumbar curve, or lordosis.... The same mechanisms are operative in pot-belly

obesity.... Even the wearing of high heels may temporarily cause the pelvis to tilt and the low back to arch enough to cause low back pain.... Difference in the length of the legs or flexion contracture of one hip or knee may tilt the pelvis sideways and require compensatory curvature of the spine to bring the head over the center of gravity (52,53).

WORKS CITED

Bourdillon, J.F. *Spinal Manipulation.* London: William Heinemann, 1982.

Cardoso, Bruce, DC, et al. *Chiropractic Technician's Program.* Vancouver, Washington: Pettibon Bio-Mechanics Institute, 1983.

Cherry, Laurence. "A Hospital Is No Place for a Sick Person to Be." *Discover* October 1985: 96-101.

CiRullo Jr., Bernard L., DC. *The Ethics of Chiropractic.* San Bernardino, California: Academy of Life, 1979.

Clark, Matt and Deborah Witherspoon. "Still Too Many Caesareans?" *Newsweek* 31 December 1984: 70.

Cyriax, James, MD. *The Slipped Disc.* London: Gower Press, 1971.

Dorland's Illustrated Medical Dictionary. Philadelphia: W.B. Saunders, 1974

Etziony, M.B., MD. *The Physician's Creed.* Springfield, Illinois: Charles C. Thomas, 1973.

Gielow, Vern. *Old Dad Chiro,* Davenport, Iowa: Bawden Bros., 1985.

Gilbert, Susan. "Hospital-Born Infections." *Science Digest* May 1985: 34.

Gregg Medical Standard Shorthand Manual and Dictionary. New York: McGraw Hill, 1953

Hole, Jr., John W. *Human Anatomy and Physiology.* Dubuque, Iowa: William C. Brown, 1984.

Imrie, David, MD. *Goodbye Backache.* New York: Arco, 1983.

Katz, Jane, Ed D. *Swimming For Total Fitness.* Garden City, New York: Dolphin Books/Doubleday, 1981.

Keim, Hugo A., MD. *How to Care for Your Back.* Englewood Cliffs, New Jersey: Prentice-Hall, 1981.

Lawrence, D. Baloti. *Massage Techniques.* New York: Putnam, 1986.

Leach, Robert A., DC. *The Chiropractic Theories: A Synopsis of Scientific Research.* Baltimore: Williams and Wilkins, 1986.

Naisbitt, John. *Megatrends.* New York: Warner, 1982.

Nieman, David C., DHSc. *The Sports Medicine Fitness Course,* Palo Alto, California: Bull, 1986.

Nelson, Harry and Anne C. Roark. "Health Care Crisis: Less for More." *Los Angeles Times* 7 April 1985, Sec. A, 1.

Newspaper Enterprise Association. *The World Almanac and Book of Facts 1986.* New York: Newspaper Enterprise Assoc., 1985.

O'Malley, C.D. *Andreas Vesalius of Brussels: 1514-1564.* Berkeley: University of California Press, 1965.

Palmer, B.J., DC. *Chiropractic Philosophy Vol. V,* Davenport, Iowa: Palmer School of Chiropractic, 1916.

Palmer, B.J., DC. *Chiropractic Philosophy: Booklet #1.* Davenport, Iowa: Palmer School of Chiropractic, [n.d.].

Palmer, D.D., DC. *The Chiropractor's Adjustor.* Portland, Oregon: Portland Printing House, 1910.

Petersen, William F., MD. *Hippocratic Wisdom.* Springfield, Illinois: Charles C. Thomas, 1946.

Pettibon, Burl R., DC. and Donald D. Harrison DC. *Chiropractic: The Correction of Abnormal Spinal Angles and the Removal of the Piezoelectric and Streaming Potential Effects of Nerve Interference.* Tacoma, Washington: Pettibon and Associates, 1978.

Pettibon, Burl R., DC. and Donald D. Harrison DC. *Spinal Biomechanics and the Pettibon Spinal Model.* Vancouver, Washington: Pettibon Bio-Mechanics Institute, [n.d.].

Pettibon, DC Burl R. and Donald D. Harrison DC. *Pettibon Spinal Biomechanics: Theory and Implications.* Vancouver, Washington: Pettibon Bio-Mechanics Institute, 1981.

Pope, Malcolm H., PhD., John W. Frymower MD, and Gunnar Andersson MD. *Occupational Low Back Pain.* New York: Praeger Special Studies, 1984.

Root, Leon MD, and Thomas Kiernan. *Oh, My Aching Back.* New York: David McKay Co., 1973.

Rowe, M. Laurens, MD. *Backache at Work.* Fairport, New York: Perinton Press, 1983.

Steinman, Marion. *American Medical Association Book of Backcare.* New York: Random House, 1982.

U.S. Bureau of the Census, *Statistical Abstract of the United States: 1986.* Washington D.C., 1986.

Venzmer, Gerhard. *5000 Years of Medicine.* New York: Taplinger, 1968.

INDEX

A

B

C

D

U

V

W

X

Y

SHARE *THE REAL TRUTH ABOUT HEALTH* WITH FAMILY, FRIENDS, EMPLOYEES, AND CO-WORKERS.

THE REAL TRUTH ABOUT HEALTH is brought to life through audience participation workshops presented by author William J. Nelson and his team of specialists. Your business, club, organization, school or church group can benefit from this lively and engaging program. Each workshop is custom tailored. Impactful information is presented through individually designed demonstrations and group interaction.

- Learn spinal self-maintenance
- Discover common sense operation of your body
- Experience proper posture, walking, lifting
- Discuss your occupation's effect on your body
- Integrate healthy behavior into your lifestyle
- Clarify self-care issues
- Communicate with your doctor more effectively
- Get more results from your efforts

A PROGRAM TO REDUCE YOUR HEALTH CARE COSTS
For more information, check box on form below

For additional copies of *THE REAL TRUTH ABOUT HEALTH,* send form to Kaptur Press, 1548-D Adams Ave., Costa Mesa, CA 92626

Send ______ copy(s) @ $13.95 each $____________

CA residents add 6% sales tax $____________

Shipping: First book $1.50
Additional books $1.00 each $____________

TOTAL ENCLOSED $____________

MAKE CHECK PAYABLE TO KAPTUR PRESS

NAME ____

ADDRESS ____

CITY ____________________________ STATE ________

ZIP CODE ____

☐ SEND WORKSHOP INFORMATION
☐ SEND QUANTITY BOOK PRICING
